CRYSTALS FOR HEALING

Discover the Power of Crystal Energy Vibrations to Heal

(How to Heal, Balance Chakras and Increase Your Spiritual Energy)

Edna Nelson

Published by Harry Barnes

Edna Nelson

All Rights Reserved

Crystals for Healing: Discover the Power of Crystal Energy Vibrations to Heal (How to Heal, Balance Chakras and Increase Your Spiritual Energy)

ISBN 978-1-7751430-4-8

All rights reserved. No part of this guide may be reproduced in any form without permission in writing from the publisher except in the case of brief quotations embodied in critical articles or reviews.

Legal & Disclaimer

The information contained in this book is not designed to replace or take the place of any form of medicine or professional medical advice. The information in this book has been provided for educational and entertainment purposes only.

The information contained in this book has been compiled from sources deemed reliable, and it is accurate to the best of the Author's knowledge; however, the Author cannot guarantee its accuracy and validity and cannot be held liable for any errors or omissions. Changes are periodically made to this book. You must consult your doctor or get professional medical advice before using any of the suggested remedies, techniques, or information in this book.

Upon using the information contained in this book, you agree to hold harmless the Author from and against any damages, costs, and expenses, including any legal fees potentially resulting from the application of any of the information provided by this guide. This disclaimer applies to any damages or injury caused by the use and application, whether directly or indirectly, of any advice or information presented, whether for breach of contract, tort, negligence, personal injury, criminal intent, or under any other cause of action.

You agree to accept all risks of using the information presented inside this book. You need to consult a professional medical practitioner in order to ensure you are both able and healthy enough to participate in this program.

Table of Contents

INTRODUCTION 1

CHAPTER 1: ORIGIN OF CRYSTAL HEALING 3

CHAPTER 2: 48 TYPES OF CRYSTALS AND THEIR HEALING MEANING 14

CHAPTER 3: CRYSTALS, CHAKRAS, AND THE HUMAN ENERGY FIELD 26

CHAPTER 4: APOPHYLLITE 39

CHAPTER 5: USING QUARTZ CRYSTALS AND ATTRACTION LAW 55

CHAPTER 6: HOW CAN I USE CRYSTALS TO REDUCE STRESS FROM WORK? 86

CHAPTER 7: TIPS FOR SELECTING HEALING CRYSTALS 94

CHAPTER 8: CHOOSING HEALING CRYSTALS FOR ANXIETY AND STRESS 98

CHAPTER 9: CRYSTAL CARE 128

CHAPTER 10: HEALING WITH CRYSTALS 142

CHAPTER 11: 20 POWERFUL CRYSTALS AND THEIR HEALING PROPERTIES 173

CONCLUSION... **191**

Introduction

Crystals and special gemstones also known as rare gems, have been around for thousands of years. From ancient people and cultures to modern day spiritual-seekers and engagers, crystals have been recognized for their unique healing properties. Crystals are metaphysical entities; they have an energy field similar to our own. OK, they may not feel, move about or breathe and live like we do, but they are still conscious and aware on a level. You see, crystals emit subtle vibrations and unique frequencies of energy. These frequencies, vibrations and energies are determined by the unique type of crystal and these are further influenced by astrological entities and forces in the earth. **As above so below** applies very much to the crystal queen and kingdom. We can tune into the crystal's unique energy for healing, wholeness and integration.

Crystal healing or simply using crystals in everyday life has a number of different applications. Firstly, crystals can be used in meditation for health, to develop a positive mindset, to balance and clear emotions, and to revitalize your spirit. They can be used in special culinary creations such as crystal water, gem essences or gem water, in which you absorb the healing effects of the unique and specific gemstone which has been immersed in the water. Crystals can also be used in divination, as protection stones like pendants and jewelry, and in more advanced healing and self-development techniques. They can be carried around to bring some joy and positivity into your life, or utilized in crystal treatments (for self or others!). In truth, the uses and benefits of crystals are so vast that one small and individual gem can create a world of magic and a reality of wonder...

Chapter 1: Origin Of Crystal Healing

Ancient civilizations around the world used crystals both as ornaments and functionally for medicine, rituals, healing, meditation, protection, offerings, and currency.

One of the earliest references is in the Enûma Eliš. This is known as the Creation Epic, recorded in Old Babylonian, and references the great god Marduk heading out for battle. Between his lips he carries an amulet made of red stone for protection. These clay tablets date back to 7th century BCE, but some believe that the composition of the text dates back to the Bronze Age or early time of Hammurabi (c. 1792 – 1750 BCE). The reports throughout history are plentiful.

Paleolithic gravesites in Switzerland and Belgium yielded jewelry made of jet. The Bishop of Rennes in the 11th century claimed that agate would make the wearer agreeable and persuasive. Ecclesiastical rings in the 12th century favored sapphires. Historical documents from Ancient Sumerians of Mesopotamia reference the use of crystals in magic formulas. Ancient Egyptians used lapis lazuli, emerald, turquoise, and clear quartz in their jewelry for protection and health and constructed healing elixirs made of crystals. In Ancient China, Chinese emperors were buried in jade armor. China and South America also used it as a kidney healing stone.

In 1880, two French Physicists, Jacques and Pierre Curie, made a scientific discovery. The Piezoelectric Effect revealed something that generations already knew because they felt drawn to use them: crystals emit forces. In short, piezoelectricity is the electrical charge that accumulates in crystals (also in bones and DNA) when subjected to pressure. With their knowledge of pyroelectricity and their understanding of crystal structures, they could predict crystal behavior and demonstrated this using crystals like quartz, tourmaline, and topaz. This was one of the first times that crystal energy was confirmed scientifically. But it wasn't the last.

Healing Crystal Trough History

Crystals and gemstones have played a part in all religions. They are mentioned throughout the Bible, in the Koran and many other religious texts. The origin of birthstones is the breastplate of Aaron, or the "High Priest's Breastplate", as mentioned in the book of Exodus. In the Koran, the 4th Heaven is composed of carbuncle (garnet). The Kalpa Tree, which represents an offering to the gods in Hinduism, is said to be made entirely of precious stone and a Buddhist text from the 7th century describes a diamond throne situated near the Tree of Knowledge (the neem tree under which Siddhartha meditated). On this throne a thousand Kalpa Buddhas reposed. The

Kalpa Sutra, in Jainism, speaks of Harinegamesi the divine commander of the foot troops who seized 14 precious stones, cleansed them of their lesser qualities and retained only their finest essence to aid his transformations.

There is also an ancient sacred lapidary treatise, the Ratnapariksha of Buddhabhatta. Some sources state that it is Hindu but it is most likely Buddhist. The date is uncertain, but it is probably from the 6th Century. In this treatise diamonds figure highly, as the king of gemstones and are ranked according to caste. The Sanskrit word for diamond, vajra, is also the word for the Hindu goddess Indra's thunderbolt and diamonds are often associated with thunder. The ruby was also highly revered. It represented an inextinguishable flame, and was purported to preserve both the physical and mental health of the wearer. The treatise lists many other gemstones and their properties.

The beginning of crystal healing

In 1609 Anselmus de Boot, court physician to Rudolf II of Germany, suggested that any virtue a gemstone has is due to the presence of good or bad angels. The good angels would confer a special grace to the gems, but the bad angels would tempt people into believing in the stone itself, and not in God's gifts bestowed on it. He goes on to name certain stones as helpful, and put other's qualities down simply to superstition. Later in the same century, Thomas Nicols expressed in his 'Faithful Lapidary' that gems, as inanimate objects, could not possess the effects claimed in the past. Thus, in the Age of Enlightenment, the use of precious stones for healing and protection began to fall from favour in Europe.

In the early part of the 19th century, a number of interesting experiments were conducted to demonstrate the effects of stones on subjects who believed themselves to be clairvoyant. In one case, the subject claimed to feel not only physical and emotional changes when touched with various stones, but also to experience smells and tastes.

New Age movement and rediscovery of gemstone use

In the 1980s, with the advent of the New Age culture, the use of crystals and gemstones began to re-emerge as a healing method. Much of the practise was drawn from old traditions, with more information gained by experimentation and channelling. Books by Katrina Rafaell in the 80s, and Melody and Michael Gienger in the 90s, helped to popularise the use of crystals.

These days there are a large number of books available on the subject, and crystals frequently feature in magazine and newspaper articles. Crystal therapy crosses the boundaries of religious and spiritual beliefs. It is no longer viewed as the domain of alternative culture, but as an acceptable and more mainstream complimentary therapy, and many colleges now offer it as a qualification subject.

Crystal healing is more a type of complementary treatment. In other words, it's used to compliment traditional medical treatment. If for example a person was being treated for cancer or some other serious type of illness, crystal energy healing could be used in a bid to enhance or boost the treatment being administered. In that sort of scenario, crystal therapy would focus on making the patient's body more responsive and receptive, and it would likewise focus on improving the patient's general frame of mind.

Even though crystal healing is often used in cases such as the one mentioned above, it's more often used to treat and cure emotional problems such as depression, anxiety, and so on. It can also be used for treating things like low self esteem, lack of confidence, and even a range of sexual issues. So, how exactly does this intriguing type of treatment work?

The Power of Crystals

While I'm not going to attempt to explain all the technicalities regarding crystals, I will point out the fact that man has long since been aware of the power of crystals, and the fact that crystals are able to harness and influence energy.

Although no longer in use medicinally, gemstones continued to hold meaning. Until recently, jet was popularly worn by those in mourning, and garnet was often worn in times of war. There is a tradition in a local family here in southwest England: every female descendent wears an antique moonstone necklace for her wedding, which has been in the family for generations. It was only recently that one family member realised this was a fertility symbol.

Many tribal cultures have continued the use of gemstones in healing until very recently, if not through to the present day. The Zuni tribe in New Mexico make stone fetishes, which represent animal spirits. These were ceremonially 'fed' on powdered turquoise and ground maize. Beautiful inlaid fetishes are still made to sell, and are very collectable artefacts or sculptures, although the spiritual practise surrounding them is no longer much in use. Other Native American tribes still hold precious stones, especially turquoise, sacred. Both Aborigines and Maoris have traditions regarding stones and healing or spiritual practise, some of which they share with the rest of the world, while some knowledge still kept private within their communities.

It is interesting to note that there are many examples of gemstones meaning similar things to different cultures, even when there has been absolutely no interaction between these cultures, and no opportunity for crossover. Jade was considered to be a kidney healing stone by the ancient Chinese, and also Aztec and Mayan civilisations, turquoise has been worn to give strength and health all over the world, and jaspers have almost always conferred both strength and calm.

In traditional Indian medicine, seven chakras are believed to be present on the surface of the human body, running in a straight line down the center of the body, parallel to the spine. These seven chakras can be described as being energy centers, with each center being responsible for a certain region of the body.

Crown Chakra

3rd Eye Chakra

Throat Chakra

Heart Chakra

Solar Plexus Chakra

Sacral Chakra

Root/Base Chakra

It is believed that if/when one or more of these chakras are blocked, the resultant disruption to the natural flow of energy causes health related problems, whether physical or emotional. In order to restore inner harmony, any blockages must be opened, and this is essentially what crystal healing aims to achieve.

Chapter 2: 48 Types Of Crystals And Their Healing Meaning

In order to make optimal use of your crystals, it is important for you to be aware of each healing stone's meanings. A healing outcome manifests itself within each crystal in a different manner. Each crystal has a different intensity and a different level of vibrations. You need to be aware of the stone's healing meaning in order to determine which type is necessary in your life and to use it for inner peace.

Agate: Agate symbolizes strength and courage. It helps to tone your mind and body by establishing a stable emotional and physical state. It works to eliminate negativity from your entire being including the mind, spirit and body. Skin and digestive diseases can be healed using this stone.

Amethyst: Amethyst represents pure spirituality and intuition. It helps individuals to calm their mind. Disorders such as insomnia and stress are reduced significantly using its healing powers. It also strengthens immunity and offers a cleansing effect on the respiratory system and organs.

Ametrine: Ametrine symbolizes optimism. It works as an amazing cleanser. Long term illnesses such as depression and fatigue can be treated using this stone. It also helps in reducing stress and headaches.

Apophyllitie: Apophyllitie is used for the recognition of truth. It helps individuals to discharge suppressed emotions and invoke deep relaxation and Reiki healing. It works as a defense against anxiety and fear and helps to treat other problems such as Asthma.

Aragonite Sputnick: The Aragonite Sputnick stone aids in patience and reliability. The healing powers of Aragonite are used to help with spasms and twitches in the nerves and muscles. It also strengthens the body by healing bones and discs.

Aquamarine: Clarity and purification in the body is induced by Aquamarine stones. Fluid retention can be controlled and nerves can be calmed using this crystal. The crystal is also used for treating sore throats and strengthening the kidneys, pituitary glands and thyroid gland.

Blue Lase Agate: Purification and communication are symbolically represented with blue lase agate. These stones offer powerful healing energies for your throat and aid in better fluid retention. Issues with blocked nervous systems and shoulder tension are also solved using the stone. Finally, bone diseases such as arthritis can be healed using this crystal in conjunction with lowering of body temperatures.

Blue Quartz: Blue quartz is used to create calmness and harmony, and it focuses extensively on stress reduction and elimination of negativity from the body, mind and spirit. This crystal can also aid in healing the throat as well.

Clear Calcite: Clear Calcite amplifies and offers a cleansing effect, and it is used for strengthening teeth, joints and bones. Toxins from organs can also be removed and other skin conditions and blood clotting difficulties can be healed. Overall, immune system becomes fortified stress is reduces through use of this stone.

Golden Calcite: Golden Calcite brings joy and lightheartedness to the user. Its healing powers include improved digestion and increased metabolism. It is also used for strengthening bones and joints and healing connective tissue and other skin related issues.

Carnelian: Carnelian evokes warmth and joy. It improves blood quality and circulation, and it stimulates the metabolism. Other healing effects include tissue regeneration and kidney and pancreas improvement.

Celestitie: Celestitie focuses on uplifting of the spirit and incorporating positivity. Eye and ear disorders and general body pain can be treated by this stone. Toxins are eliminated, bones are strengthened, and chronic tensions are released.

Chevron Amethyst: Chevron Amethyst brings about spirituality and intuition. The organs are harmonized and immune system is stimulated.

Citrine: Citrine revitalizes and cleanses. The stone helps the digestive system, reduces internal infections, and alleviates fatigue. Symptoms related to menstrual and menopausal cycles are also aided.

Clear Quartz: Clear Quartz is used to provide clarity to, and awareness of, your thoughts. The stone has powerful energies that offer healing for most conditions, and it is often used for energizing purposes.

Desert Rose: Desert Rose creates possibility. This healing stone aligns the spinal column and promotes flexibility. It also calms the nerves and helps with disorders such as epilepsy.

Epidote: Epidote is used to promote recovery and regeneration, generally through emotional uplifting and elimination of sadness. It is mainly used in post-illness states.

Fluorite: Fluorite is used to promote focus and protection. It strengthens one's capacity for understanding and helps reduce negative energies and stress while purifying and cleansing the body.

Green Aventurine: Green Aventurine invokes emotional tranquility by helping to reduce stress and anxiety. It is used for muscle stimulation and bone-related healing, and it helps to remedy sleep disorders.

Green Jade: Green Jade balances emotions. It is used for strengthening the immune system and improving one's heart and kidneys. Generally, it has a cleansing effect on the organs and blood. Other healing properties include assistance in fertility and relief from menstrual or menopausal symptoms.

Hermatite: Hermatite promotes energy and vitality and enhances stress resistance. The stone helps with circulatory issues, in turn improving the flow of oxygen across the body, stimulating glands, and activating the spleen and gallbladder.

Jasper Red: Jasper Red is used to stimulate blood flow and digestive systems, and it focuses circulation on sexual organs.

Leumarian Seeded Crystal: Leumarian seeded crystal aids in removing diseases generally by opening new energy channels in organs.

Labradorite: Labradorite helps one to find spiritual connection. It helps to balance hormones, lower blood pressure, and treat eye and brain disorders.

Pyrite Cube: The pyrite cube offers protection, and it is used to seek relief from anxiety and frustration. It also improves brain functioning and oxygenation and blood circulation.

Petrified Wood: Petrified wood promotes inner harmony. It improves blood circulation, helps treat arthritis and blood clots, improves appetites and soothes nerves.

Rose Quartz: The beautiful rose crystal promotes love and peace. It strengthens the human heart and blood circulation through treating chest and respiratory issues, and it increases fertility.

Selenite: Selenite allows for clarity and enhances willpower through the soothing of nerves.

Separtian: Using separtian enhances communication abilities and helps one uplift and understand the spirit.

Shungite: Also known as the wonder stone, shungite restores all that is useful, and eliminates all that is harmful, to the individual.

Shiva Lingam: Shiva lingham helps stimulate the electrical flow of bodies and is useful for treating infertility and cramps.

Smokey Quartz: Smokey quartz dissipates negativity and blocked energies while enhancing awareness and focus.

Spirit Quartz: The uplifting spirit quartz facilitates in cellular and spiritual healing that helps during times of grief.

Tourmaline Black: Tourmaline black is a highly supportive crystal with healing powers sleep disorders. It improves the immune system, offers pain relief, and aids the colon, legs, spinal column and kidneys.

Tibetan Quartz: The Tibetan quartz stone promotes spiritual protection and help heals the brain and nervous system. It removes negativity and negative electromagnetic energies and offers spiritual growth.

Tiger Iron: Tiger iron, the crystal of manifestation, has potential to enhance an individual's physical energy. It helps overcome fatigue and improves circulation and blood cell counts.

Tiger Eye: Tiger eye stones encourage personal power. It helps balance emotions and reduces headaches. It also improves the reproductive system and relieves asthma attacks. Finally, it also enhances night vision.

Botswana Agate: The Botswana agate focuses on creativity and solutions. The stone improves the nervous system and strengthens broken bones.

Angel Wing/Alunite: The angel wing is used to balance negative and positive energies. It enhances and improves creativity and mental stability.

Apache Tears: Apache tears stone is the most helpful in times of grief. It helps the individual release negative emotions.

Apatite: The amazing apatite stone helps improve intuitive awareness, intellect and imagination which results in better decision making.

Aqua Aura: The stunning aqua aura crystal is useful for increasing psychic and conscious awareness of an individual.

Abalone: Also known as sea ears, Abalone helps to stimulate instinctive feelings. It clears fear, sorrow and other negative emotions from the heart. Psychic development is also aided along with intuition.

Kansas Pop Rock: The Kansas pop rock heals the body by releasing blockages and clots.

Kinoite: Kinoite stones improve communication, aid psychic disorders, and promote truth.

Kunzite: The kunzite crystal helps reduce stress, making it amazing in for managing grief and heart conditions.

Variscite: Also known as "True Worry Stone," variscite stones are helpful for releasing physical and mental tensions. It also helps the nervous system and kidneys.

Diopside: Diopside heals the mind, calms anxiety, and assists with learning power.

Chapter 3: Crystals, Chakras, And The Human Energy Field

How Do I Use Crystals for Healing?

Your body is made up of energy centers called chakras. The major chakras run down the length of your body from the top of your head to your sacrum. They are situated in key positions and govern body functions exclusive to each part. For instance, the heart chakra on your chest affects your ability to give and receive love while the throat chakra on your neck influences your ability to express yourself. Think of chakras as small wheels constantly rotating, drawing in and giving off energy from the universe. When the wheels are blocked, they cease to turn. When they do, the body part associated with that chakra malfunctions. Hence, when your throat chakra is blocked, you may find it hard to communicate with others.

This inability to speak your mind will eventually diminish your emotional and mental wellbeing. At the same time, the inability of the clogged chakra to emit and draw in energy will bring about physical symptoms affecting the neck. This disruption in your body's balance will cause the other chakras to overcompensate, causing physical strain as well as imbalances in one's personality. For instance, an overactive heart chakra that's trying to compensate for an underactive throat chakra will cause an individual to be exceedingly emotional and make him an easy prey for people who choose to take advantage.

The worst part is, with the whole balance disrupted, it's only a matter of time before the excessive work takes its toll and disease starts to manifest in various systems of the body. It's no rocket science. Just think of how many individuals who keep their emotions bottled up (blocked throat chakra) end up suffering from cardiovascular diseases (overworked heart chakra).

The solution for such cases will be to heal the blocked chakra to restore the overall balance. As it is, one of the easiest ways to use crystals for healing is to simply lay them on the affected chakras. That said, you can't just pick a pretty stone and lay it on your body. Certain chakras respond more effectively to certain crystals. The different chakras consist of their unique colors. For the throat chakra, it's blue. As a rule (though not a strict one), a chakra will respond positively to a crystal, which is of the same color. That's because they possess the same frequency, thus, blue crystals like turquoise are recommended for the throat chakra. The turquoise will heal the throat chakra through entrainment. That is, the throat chakra will automatically align itself with the turquoise (object with the more powerful frequency) then restore its harmony.

Additionally, you may also use this method to activate dormant chakras. For a lot of people, the brow chakra, also known as the third-eye chakra is tightly shut. Thankfully, with the use of the right crystals, you can awaken this chakra and consequently, awaken your innate psychic abilities.

What is the Human Energy Field and What is its Connection with the Chakras?

As all beings are made up of energy, it is through the human energy field that we are connected with other existing beings, with other existing energies. The human energy field, also known as the "aura", encompasses and permeates your body. Within it, you'll find the energetic aspects of each of your body parts and body functions. The human energy field, therefore, triggers and supports all your bodily functions. More than that, it contains everything that you experience - from your physical senses to your thoughts and emotions.

Energy flows through your aura through networks called nadis. Nadis are also made up of energy. The points through which these networks cross are your energy distribution hubs or your chakras. As such, each human energy field level has a consistent chakra. It is from and with the Universal Energy Field that the chakras receive and exchange energy.

Crystals for the Different Human Energy Field Levels and Chakras

Etheric Level

This is the surrounding substance which your physical body is formed.

Corresponding Chakra:

Base Chakra

The first chakra is situated at the base of your spine and is also called the Root Chakra. It governs your survival instinct and your ability to preserve yourself. Its energy is focused on keeping your grounded and stable. The base chakra's color is red and as such, you can heal it by using red crystals like garnet, hematite, and bloodstone.

Emotional Level

This fluid energy level governs emotions particularly those related with your perception of yourself.

Corresponding Chakra:

Sacral Chakra

Located below your navel is your second chakra, which governs your sexuality and your reproductive abilities. Its color is orange. The crystals that work best with this energy center are orange calcite, orange zincite, red jasper, red and brown aventurine and carnelian.

Mental Level

In this level, you'll find the blueprint of your logical brain. That includes views that are positive and beliefs that are destructive.

Corresponding Chakra:

Solar Plexus Chakra

The third chakra is found at your solar plexus and its color is yellow. It governs your intellect, will and = ambition. Use crystals like yellow jasper, citrine, golden calcite, amber, topaz and yellow sapphire to heal this energy center.

Astral Level

This multi-colored energy layer is concerned with your experiences and relationships in this life and in the ones before.

Corresponding Chakra:

Heart Chakra

On the center of your chest is your fourth chakra. Its color is pink and green. It governs your capacity for love, compassion, and emotional balance. The best stones for this chakra are emerald, green calcite, jade, green tourmaline, malachite, aventurine, moonstone and rose quartz.

Template Level

This level is the entryway between your body and your mind. This layer cradles the blueprint for your creative power.

Corresponding Chakra:

Throat Chakra

Above your collarbone sits your fifth chakra, which controls your power to speak your personal truth. Its color, as mentioned, is blue. Apart from the blue turquoise, you may also use blue lace agate, angelite, sapphire, aquamarine, blue calcite, blue topaz, and blue kyanite for healing.

Celestial Level

This is the level where you develop your consciousness. The celestial level is that which connects you with the higher realms.

Corresponding Chakra:

Brow Chakra

Nestled in the medulla is your third eye chakra. The focus of its energy is on spiritual awareness and intuition. This energy center governs your psychic ability and extrasensory perception. Your sixth chakra's color is indigo. The proper stones to use for healing are amethyst, sodalite, azurite, and lapis lazuli.

Causal Level

This is the level which encompasses all the other layers. Think of it as the sheath which holds all the fabrics of your being together. This is where you can recognize the faultlessness of "what is".

Corresponding Chakra:

Crown Chakra

The seventh chakra is found at the top of your head. Its colors are violet and white. It is the energy center, which is concerned with your connection with the divine, cosmic consciousness and spiritual wisdom. If you are deficient in this area, use crystals like amethyst, quartz, diamond, clear calcite and white topaz.

Chakra Balancing

If you feel like you are out of tune (low spirits, unproductive, confused with life, restless), then you can balance your chakras by doing the following at home on a regular basis.

Obtain one crystal for each of the corresponding chakras. This means you need to have crystals with colors that represent the entire spectrum of the rainbow.

Next, you need to cleanse your crystals to get rid of negative energy. This will be discussed in detail in the succeeding chapters.

Then, cleanse your healing space (ex. your room, or anywhere you feel safe and comfortable).

Assume a comfortable supine lying position.

Tap your thymus for 30 seconds.

Begin with your base chakra. Lay the corresponding stone (ex. garnet) on that area.

Then, lay the corresponding stone (ex. carnelian) on your sacral chakra.

Do the same for your solar plexus chakra, heart chakra, then throat chakra.

Proceed to placing the right healing crystal on your brow chakra. Finally, lay the corresponding stone at the base of your crown.

Maintain your position for half an hour.

During this time, imagine the colors of the crystals glowing.

In your mind's eye, witness how each chakra glows in response to the corresponding stone.

Then, feel the wheels of your seven major chakras turning. All of them are in sync. As you breathe in, they are absorbing energy from the crystals. As you breathe out, the chakras are exhaling all the accumulated negative energies.

Once you're done, remove first the crystal on the crown chakra. Then remove the one from your brow chakra.

Once you're done removing the crystal from your base chakra, you may take a glass of water or go for a walk so you can ground yourself. This way, you can even out the healing energy, which you've absorbed.

Note: More important than the crystal's unique attribute is the way you feel about it. You need to feel a personal resonance or connection with the crystal. We are like strings in two violins. When you pluck a string, the string from the other violin with the same note will respond. When you're purchasing a crystal, opt for the one which calls outto you.

Chapter 4: Apophyllite

Apophyllite is a spiritual advisor stone which carries and emits higher than average vibrational energies that serve to enhance our own, bringing feelings of peace and contentment. It is a stone that normally forms clear and colourless but sometimes contains hues of light green are believed to have the ability to purify spaces by filling them with calming energy and high-level vibrational fields. Apophyllite carries within itself the power of ancient lava flows which act upon the user's emotional energies eliminating feelings of fear and anxiety. Apophyllite's vibrational energy is first and foremost a healing energy, powerful enough to instantly dissolve stress, break and absorb negative thought patterns freeing the mind to creative thought and that which makes us happy. It is said that sitting and holding an Apophyllite stone for 30 minutes is more effective and cheaper than seeing a professional therapist. This is a stone that brings negative energies into itself so it is important to cleanse and recharge Apophyllite crystal regularly to avoid any build-up of unwanted energy. It is the perfect stone for those dealing with personal worries and past traumas that they do not wish to share with anyone else, carrying Apophyllite works wonders for those suffering from daily stress, unhelpful thought patterns. It soothes frayed nerves through its links with and activation of the Heart Chakra which in turn act to realign the body's energy field with that of the Earth. Apophyllite crystals are known to be great facilitators of out of body experiences, past life regressions and astral travel. The physical healing properties of Apophyllite are well known and it has been used to cure coughs and even Asthma and other respiratory conditions. It promotes healthy and regular skin growth making it great for healing scars, skin issues and some allergic reactions.

Colour

Clear

Sometimes carries hues of light green.

Zodiac

Aries

Capricorn

Scorpio

Planet

Mars

Saturn

Energetic Frequency

Calming

Healing

Chakras

Heart

Aquamarine

Getting its name from the Latin aqua Marinus meaning 'water of the sea' Aquamarine has long been worn by sailors for protection while on the water. This calming stone in its hues of blue and green invokes the purity and clarity of crystalline waters with deep connections to trust, truth, and revelation, which when used as a meditation aid can act as a mirror revealing the hidden meanings of reality and even our owns inner depths. Ancient seers and modern alike believe Aquamarine to be under the influence of and magnetically connected to the moon and its cycles, allowing the skilled mystic or seer to foresee coming events especially as the moon is increasing. It is thought that the moon's magnetism affects the iron oxides present within the Aquamarine and it is this process that enhances the gemstone's forecasting abilities. Aquamarine has long been associated with wisdom, openness, reasoning, and accelerated learning, it has been told that with the help of Aquamarine one can become unconquerable through learning. Its connection to the throat chakra brings about feelings of calmness, moderation, rationality and responsibility making it the perfect representation of justice. Aquamarine is the ideal talisman for those regularly involved in negotiations requiring delicacy compromise and understanding as well as for those who commonly deal with difficult or challenging individuals and has since ancient times been worn as protection by those who travel on water. Aquamarine is also known as a seeker energiser crystal which means specific energy structures that have the natural ability to align with and synchronise to the energy fields that surround the human body amplifying the universal life force that flows throughout each of us. The ancient Romans even used Aquamarine talismans to purify water, believing it to be a treasure of the mermaids, holding protective, even purifying qualities that could counteract overeating and aid in digestion, often drinking from goblets carved from Aquamarine. In modern times it is regularly worn as a pendant to reduce and sooth problems relating to the thymus gland.

Colour

Bluey/Green

Birthstone

March

Zodiac

Scorpio

Aquarius

Energetic Frequencies

Healing

Power

Protection

Chakra

The Fifth or Throat Chakra

Aragonite

Aragonite is a gemstone displaying light tan, almost brown colour hues and is found in Mexico, Morocco and Spain. It is a stone that carries strong connections to the Earth and its energy field which in turn links it primarily to the Root Chakra but also to the Crown and Sacral Chakra. Aragoniteis a crystal that promotes healthy brain functions including, memory, creativity, focus and concentration. The grounding energy emitted by Aragonite lifts the body's vibrational frequency and grounds the energetic field produced by the body's kinetic, emotional and chakra networks. When we meditate with Aragonite it centres the emotions and stabilises temperaments which in turn strengthen patience and determination. Aragonite's ability to aid self-control and discipline helps to bolster our defences against unhelpful situations and unruly people. The healing qualities of Aragonite are well known and it is believed to speed up the recovery of broken bones as well as nerve damage, exhaustion and enhance the body's ability to process calcium. Emotionally, Aragonite heals frayed nerves, lowers stress levels and sleeping with Aragonite is a well-known cure for insomnia. Aragonite simulates personal growth, carrying or wearing it can help relieve depression and support those leaving difficult situations, people or lifestyles.

Colour

Light brown

Tan

Zodiac

Capricorn

Energetic Frequencies

Healing

Nature

Transition

Chakras

Root Chakra

Crown Chakra

Sacral Chakra

Aventurine

Aventurine crystals are gemstones that contain a healthy amount of Quartz along with other mineral inclusion that acts together to give Aventurine its varying colours. These differing mineral inclusions influence not only the stone's colour but also its inherent energetic attributes, meaningful associations and healing abilities. Its name is derived from the Italian a Ventura meaning 'by chance' and is most commonly associated with luck, regularly known as the 'Stone of Opportunity'.

Green Aventurine

Green Aventurine is not just a gemstone of luck forever acting to bend chance to your favour, it is also thought to increase creative insight and heighten attention and **6th** sense perception. This miraculous gemstone works by first releasing the wearer of and purging any unhelpful and negative habits and connections, opening us up to the natural energies of the stone which then act to align and create conditions (usually through coincidences) that coincide with our needs and goals. Green Aventurine had has a long list of uses throughout the ages. In more modern times it is often worn as protection against the electromagnetic pollution that surrounds us daily and leaving a stone in a bowl of water overnight and then washing your face with it the next day has been said to cure skin conditions like acne, and eczema. Green Aventurine's healing energies help guard against heart and circulatory problems as well as eyesight issues light short-sightedness. The stones direct links with the Heart Chakras energetic aura means Green Aventurine is a fitting aid or talisman for those who suffer from a short temper, the calming influence of Green Aventurine harmonises the body's natural energy flow leaving us less susceptible to outside stresses.

Blue Aventurine

Blue Aventurine is another lucky gemstone with direct access to the Third Eye and so is known to be a very powerful mental healer as well as being great for those looking to increase their willpower and determination. By combining the elements of wind and water, Blue Aventurine exudes an influential energy of gentle rationality that steadily guides the user towards greater levels of inner strength and self-discipline. Blue Aventurine is perfect for those looking to break destructive habits like smoking and substance abuse due to its ability to bestow on the wearer the ability to take charge and stick to their decisions. It is also an exceptionally useful stone for travellers, protecting them and their luggage from problems during their journey like delays, losses, and illnesses. Blue Aventurine has a strong connection to both the Brow and Throat Chakra which partner up and combines to provide relief for those who suffer from a fiery temperament by surrounding them with gentle calming energies that deflect negative outside interferences.

Red Aventurine

Red Aventurine, otherwise known as the 'stone of manifestation through action' and gives the user's conscious the ability to break free from the ego and further strengthen their perseverance and determination. This stone is said to emanate a level-headed yet spontaneous energy that has proved incredibly useful in households where sibling rivalry is rife. The strong yet stable energetic frequencies of Red Aventurine work to firstly to clear and balance the Base Chakra, then to activate the Root or Base Chakra supercharging our self-confidence bordering on a fearlessness that propels down our desired paths. This is a stone filled with possibilities that when worn will assist any creative projects and enlighten you to amazing opportunities hidden within the everyday world.

Colour

Green

Blue

Red

Birthstone

August

Energetic Frequencies

Prosperity

Luck

Healing

Chakras

The Heart Chakra (green)

The Third Eye or Brow Chakra (blue)

The Throat Chakra (blue)

The Base or Root Chakra (red)

Barite

Barite is a crystal that has many forms and colourings. Depending on the environment in which Barite forms it can form with prismatic crystals, lamellar, and fibrous crystalline-like structures. Barite's colouring ranges from deep greens, and blues through to reds, browns, yellow, black, colourless and at times even fluorescent. Barite has been known to form in tubular concentric crystals resulting in a pattern that is similar to that of a flower; these rare barites are extremely popular among gem collectors, Reiki practitioners and healers alike. Barite was renowned by Native Americans as a ritual stone with powerful healing properties and has been valued as such ever since. Barite's natural energetic field is known to stimulate brain functions like memory recall, willpower, determination and creativity. It has also been used to enhance psychic abilities, allowing for past life regression, lucid dreaming and communication with otherworldly entities and the higher realms of consciousness. Barite is commonly used to aid the body's detoxification processes, eliminating built up toxins, environmental pollutants that accumulate in the body. As a healing stone Barite is one of the many stones that break up energetic blockages, however, carrying or wearing Barite over prolonged periods of time, months or even years will balance and maintain the natural flow of energy throughout the body's energetic and chakra networks improving health, mood and longevity. Barite has the ability to break negative thought patterns which makes it perfect for anyone suffering from emotional loss, stress and/or addiction. Barite's energy enters the chakra through the Third Eye Chakra an is one of the few stones known to actually boost the body's chakra energy or 'chi' and so is highly valued by spiritualist and those who practice both meditation and the martial arts.

Colour

Green

Blue

Red

Brown

Yellow

Black

Colourless

Birthstone

No association

Zodiac

Aquarius

Energetic Frequencies

Healing

Chakras

The Third Eye

Chapter 5: Using Quartz Crystals And Attraction Law

Millions of people worldwide have become aware of the Law of Attraction since the book was published and the movie The Secret released. In this chapter, I will discuss the fundamental tenets of the Law of Attraction and teach you another mystery: how, using quartz crystals, you can achieve even more powerful results to increase the cycle of realization promised by the Law of Attraction.

In short, the Law of Attraction says that somehow the reality we experience in our lives–our degree of happiness, success, love and wealth –depends on our thinking and emotions. Everything you think most carefully on, whether good or bad, comes into your life, which we call manifestation.

Manifestation takes place in three stages. Such steps can be used in a wide range of commercially available coaching methods and other self-enhancing, wealth and success programs: o STEP 1: Your motivation takes form in your hopes, aspirations and specific goals.

o STEP 2: The world listens to your request and keeps for you your wish in the area of opportunity.

O STEP 3: You sync yourself internally to a higher frequency that allows for your desired voice.

The chapter will discuss these steps more closely and then show you how to use quartz crystals to improve the cycle of manifestation.

Put the three steps into Practice STEP 1: decide what you want. The wishes we have and wishes show out each time, but they have to be shaped in some particular way. To meet your wishes is like searching for Google: to obtain the exact returns you need to make your query very transparent and precise. If you're searching for a Google "home," you're going to get 1.3

billion hits! This is too vague. This is far too vague. You get far fewer hits if you're searching for "House, 2 Stories, Maui, Green, less than $500,000." The thoughts and questions you send to the world must be extremely concentrated and precise. Visualize your desired result, its intent, its exact characteristics, and when you will achieve it. See the result of achieving your goal in your head, perhaps even greater than you can now imagine!

STEP 2: Believe that your query has been answered by the universe. The second step takes place without your conscious awareness, so you don't have to deal with it. Be certain that the Universe will play its part in obtaining and keeping your stated intentions as possible.

STEP 3: Align to a greater frequency. The third step is the job you must do to do what you want. So repeat, whatever you focus on, your life will attract you. If you focus on a problem that is very troubling to you, you align yourself with the negative energies of the problem instead of the problem.

Problems inevitably give us bad feelings. If you decide to concentrate on these bad feelings, you give them more energy. Fortunately, you can consciously focus on the solution or what you want to bring into your life instead of the problem. If you do that, you will notice immediately that your inner state is turning into more positive feelings. It opens up a flow of ideas and solutions. You can quickly feel that you are dealing with the problem instead of being disempowered.

It is therefore important that your inner state is constantly controlled and your thoughts and feelings balanced so that they are ALIGNED with your desires instead of in opposition to them. Negative thoughts confront and deny your true wishes. Positive thoughts and feelings stimulate your real desires. When you take this habit of tracking and adjustment and instantly substitute positive for negative, you can feel good most of the time and be able to move with strength beyond all obstacles.

In addition to their great beauty, crystals have spiritual properties that can be used to enrich your life in many fantastic ways. The potential of crystals to store information for you and serve as a focal point for your thoughts and prayers is the most appealing of these attributes.

A crystal is like a computer chip where data can be processed. And a computer chip is made of silicone, the fundamental ingredient for quartz crystals.

Crystals can help you in Step 3 to consciously align yourself with your wishes and dreams by increasing your frequency of energy, aligning you with the flow to your objectives and helping you to anchor yourself as an inner state of good.

The physical characteristics of quartz crystal quartz are the most common of the world's crystals. It is composed of silicon dioxide, one of our world's most common compounds.

This forms six-sided crystals from a milky base to a transparent edge. It is commonly found in the cluster and often in conjunction with other minerals.

The spiritual properties and uses of quartz crystal quartz are very transparent and translucent, thereby making light and visible in the material realm. This symbolizes our search for success in our internal growth and elevates our consciousness to higher levels.

The Sun (light) and Saturn (crystallization) properties are astrologically crystal quartz. It is the ideal stone to show you the path to life-affirming light, to elevate you into a more optimistic inner state, to relax your mind and to help you concentrate on what is important to you.

Quartz crystals can be used in these particular ways: a quartz crystal used in relaxation helps to calm the mind and relax. The ideal crystal structure and alignment are capable of enhancing your meditation.

o You can store your thoughts, mental pictures, and emotions with a quartz crystal and improve your connection with your dream.

o A quartz crystal mounted in front of and on the hard drive of your machine will help protect you from electrosmog.

How to clean and vacuum the crystal from old vibrations Before you can use the crystal properly, it must be cleaned to remove any old vibrations it brought to your direction. Those conflict with your positive energy connection with the crystal. You want the crystal for your purposes clean and blank.

With the aid of the four elements Earth, fire, water, and air, you can create a cleansing ritual. I prefer the following air method: 1. You sit in your hand with your stone, let your mind relax, breathe in and out.

2. Place the other hand over the crystal and feel your hands in the energy field.

3. Exhale the old traces of residual energy sharply and imagine from the crystal.

Before using your crystal, you will have produced a clear picture of your purpose and goal in your mind, as mentioned above. It is better to use a different crystal for each one of your objectives so that each time you hold it, the crystal will spark that particular vision.

The crystal must be programmed for your function or intent. This is how to do this: 1. Keep the crystal as above in both hands. Stay conscious of the crystal energy field between your two sides.

2. Reflect on your dream, purpose or target carefully. Imagine powerful simplicity in it, as if you were already living through the target. Experience the strong

emotions of accomplishment and achievement that are correlated with your goal.

3. Release your goal photo with a sharp breath.

You have now preserved this type of thinking and these emotions in the crystal. This will strengthen your field of expectation; keep you tuned to the universe and call for what you want. You also place an anchor in your energy field in the programming of your dream that will hold your unconscious mind on your vision.

Eventually, sometimes sit down and hold your crystal and imagine again how good your target will be when you achieve it. Plunge into these thoughts. This is what I regularly call "firing up" your dream. This raises the intensity and helps it to move through you.

According to the Law of Attraction, you must be available, receptive, and at the right frequency if you want to satisfy your wishes. Crystals are a strong tool to aid the manifestation cycle by allowing you to increase your intensity and stay in line with your desire.

Crystals As Feng Shui Enhancements

Amethyst Amethyst is a rare stone of love and intellect. This makes it ideal for you to be in the area of knowledge or your home's relationship, to be placed in pairs. When you study to learn new skills, you can place them next to your study books on a bookcase or a chair, or if you have a home office on your desk.

Amethyst can be used on its own or a larger display. Both the fields of knowledge and relationships in your home receive energy from the earth and try to integrate it into your show. Place amethyst crystals in a square or rectangular bowl between plants or flowers or several amethyst crystals. Create a small indoor garden and reveal amethyst crystals as the rocks in the garden.

Bloodstone Bloodstones can improve intuition and imagination and are therefore a good choice for children and the home's creativity. When Bloodstones are placed, they can be used for a small display themselves or larger decor. As the component metal supports this part of the house, it would be nice to put these crystals into a small metal container. As Bloodstone is a yin stone, then if you do not put it directly in the light, it is more comfortable for you to spread stagnant chi in darker areas of your house.

Carnelian is one of those crystals with such strength that it can be used to boost various areas of your home. Carnelian is a powerful stone, probably best known for being able to invite plenty to the house. This is why the display should be located at the entrance to your home, ideally next to your door.

It is also regarded as a rock of bravery and achievement. It can help encourage positive life decisions, drive you to excel and empower you. If you need help in any of these areas of your life, Carnelian can be very useful in your career and self-esteem. Alternatively, a bowl of Carnelian Crystals on your desk can work wonders for your business success if you have a home office and want to improve your business.

Citrine is an extremely strong crystal and can be used for many applications including Carnelian. Citrine's power is very yang and can be located in any of the yang areas of the home because of this. These are the parts of the house that are northeast, east, southeast, and south when you look at your home.

If you want to raise energy in one of these regions, Citrine crystals can provide help. Citrine crystals are stunning since their bright yellow color will truly boost energy in every room. These are especially good to have in the bathroom, which can sometimes feel a bit overlooked as a functional space. Citrine crystals have the most common and popular use as a wealth remedy as they are regarded as a stone of abundance. If you want to draw capital to home, it can be very useful to put 8 citrine crystals in your region of wealth.

My favorite treatment of wealth with citrine crystals is to put 8 crystals in a wooden box with a small note. This can be placed in your area of wealth or your most favorable area, as your Kua number governs.

Green Fluorite Green fluorites are perfect stones and one of my favorites all the time. They can help to strengthen the family area when placing the stones in the home so you can place them both in the family area of your home or your main living room. Beautiful for decoration, I prefer to use it as part of a wider décor, and I've got green fluorite rocks in my own home on a narrow wooden tray with bamboo and dark green perfumed candles.

Placing Green Fluorite can help bring balance and a common understanding when you have disharmony with your immediate or extended family. Green Fluorite is an extremely relaxing stone that can help to restore broken connections and repair conflict. Green fluorite stones cover family photos to help heal broken relationships, as they can help to promote positive energy in the household.

Hematite crystals have a very powerful yang component and can sustain and enhance energy in your home area of fame and self-esteem. Hematite can mentally enhance self-confidence, eliminate weaknesses and increase growth. When you are looking for assistance in growing your faith, placing these crystals in a small bowl together or bringing them into a larger decoration can only give you the improvement you want.

Lapis Lazuli Lapis Lazuli is a lovely stone that can be used in several ways. The energy associated with these stones is very yin and can be put in any of your home's yin areas. These include your marriage, children and imagination, supportive friends and professions.

If you want to improve and boost energies, these stones can be beneficial in any of these areas of your life. The relationship between two of these stones or helpful friends can strengthen the relationship between two people. Placing these stones in children and imagination will help to open the mind to new possibilities. The placement of these stones can lead to the development of a new business in your career field or the quest for transparency and objectivity in your career goals. Nevertheless, you use these stones in your home to enhance their beauty or to decorate them in their own right.

Red Jade Red Jade is a beautiful crystal that is possibly one of the most common crystals for enhancement. Red Jade stands for understanding, love, and friendship. If you want to improve your power in any of these fields of your life, Red Jade can be a part of your home's experience, relationship, and friends.

Rose Quartz Rose Quartz is known as unconditional love stone so if you're looking for love or want to deepen your love with your partner these crystals should be put both in the relationship zone of your home and in your bedroom. As they symbolize the love between two people, these crystals must be placed always in pairs, so if you put them alongside your bed, for example, make sure to place two glasses on both sides of the bed. You can either carry the crystals in pairs, or you can give your beloved one crystal so that you each have a half pair.

One final point you should always do so deliberately when putting crystals that sustain the energy in your home. The best way to do this is to improve the three secrets before they are mounted. To reinforce the three secrets, first of all, you should imagine the outcome that you want to achieve when the crystals are put, then say loudly what you want before taking a few moments of quiet reflection at last. Keep the crystals in your left hand while you are in the field where you are going to place them.

Energy Healing

What is healing energy? What is healing energy?

Positioning of hands, also known as energy treatments, energy therapy, bioenergy therapy, biofield therapy and energy, encourages cures by improving the flow of energy and changing the body's aura. This advancement of the flow of aura energy supports the body's self-healing ability.

Laying hands is an ancient way of healing that returns to our lives in a revival of ancient understandings. People all over the world learn how to feel energy, move energy and rediscover energy healing treatments.

The use of energy fields for healing implies that a magnetic field is produced strong enough to create changes in the body without damage, and that field should be sufficiently optimized for treating particular disease as treatment with a broad frequency spectrum is not adequate.

Vibrational or hand-held healing can restore human health and harmony on four planes: IS physically and spiritually ALL OTHER KIND OF HEALING?

There isn't! No there isn't!

All that remains is energy, so each healing requires energy, although most healing methods are only physically concentrated.

Energy healing works across the energy level of our being and affects the physical, psychological, mental and spiritual aspects from there.

Energy healing is therefore a holistic method of healing because it examines the energy the body composes, complements the body and its emotions and embraces other methods of healing.

Vibrational heals use pure energy to treat people who affects the energy system acting as a kind of wave-guide to redirect or reorient the subtle energies affected.

Energy Healing works by laying on hands and is only a part of a broader field called Energy Medicine, which uses crystals, herbs, sound or control of mind.

Many healers like to use crystals or other devices to generate power-healing energy, but energy-healing is more often than not generated by the contact of the healer with the healing in an energetic stage. (Excellent energy therapy examples are the vibratory medicine of Richard Gerber and the energie medicine of James Oschman.) THE HUMAN ENERGY FIELDS The physical body in the mirror is not the one we have. There is also an energy field, called The Aura, around us. The physical body is our densest energy expression and we sometimes call many other bodies The subtle bodies There are many different descriptions of the aura of our body.

There are also other essential energy centers called The Chakras where important energy exchanges are carried out and which are often affected by energy healing.

What is Science? Such knowledge is acquired in the Western civilizing world by the' test and error method' or' scientific method' but this is not the only way to gain knowledge or I might say that the' scientific method' only acquires knowledge from the information provided by our senses.

"Scientific method" can show only what one or more of our five senses experience (we say "seeing is believe"). But there are those who can perceive by a higher sense perception. But it is also found that the observer affects the observing entity through the act of observation so that in another kind of energy field our observer requires something that happens.

And modern science makes daily discoveries of new methods of healing, consistent with the concept of manipulating the human energy field with other energies (sound, heats, etc.) Very few scientists are sure to take up the idea of energy healing, but work has begun to show that healing has an effect. Hereby I shall list only one, but in the references below you can read about the others.

A SCIENTIFIC AND Study The following experiment showed that non-contact therapists in the energy field of blindfolded subjects could cause significant changes.

A man was isolated behind a divider and his finger was taken from a conductivity picture (or Kirlian).

The testing person drew a card with the words "brighter" written (he was the only one in the room to see the card), so he went around the test subject without touching him, in an attempt to make the conductivity picture of the test subject more vivid.

The practicer moved his hands around the test subject for the following three minutes to make the conductivity picture of the text less clear, and another photograph was taken.

The photos showed clearly that when he tried to do so, the practitioner successfully increased energy and then decreased the intensity of the conductivity of the subjects, without touching him.

The brighter and smoother images seen after the experiment indicated not only that the energy of the test subject changed, but that an effective therapy was applied.

What does the Science know about the human organisms?

These fields of energy are quite measurable and well-known biophysical mechanisms can account for the observed phenomena.

We all know that the human body has electrical fields, which can be measured by techniques like EMG, EEG and EKG, without the production and receipt of electrical signals by the body.

Natural Crystals and Stones Metaphysical Qualities and Uses

Over the ages, the mystical properties of rocks, more aptly known as minerals, have intrigued people from all over the world.

Minerals promote healing, especially in their crystalline form, based on the property of sympathetic vibration or resonance. We have very common resonance points with one of our seven main energy centers (chakras). The colors of the stones appear to affect the features of the vibrations. The colors are more or less similar to the seven charcas, which also coincide with the seven rainbow colours. (Crown chakra-purple, blast chakra-indigo, chakra thorn-blue, chakra of the heart-green, plexus of the moon-red), chakra of the saints-orange, and chakra of the foundation-red). The resonant frequencies generate an electromagnetic field.

If we believe that all humans are electromagnetic and have weaves of energies (human aura) beyond their physical shells, it follows, naturally, that the electromagnetic resonance of minerals and crystals can influence them.

Increased disharmony of thoughts, diseases and diseases have been attributed to irregular energy flows within the subtle (non-physical), etheric, and physical bodies; thus, prolonged exposure to positive stone vibration can produce a healing effect. Beyond their healing effects, minerals always guard against negative effects and give us good luck.

Amulets and Talisman to drive spirits back.

Some stones, particularly those of celestial origins, seem to be able to drive away unwanted or negative energy. These are stones that can prevent evil spirits from being formed from the meteorite group— tektite, moldavites, iron and nickel meteorites. If they are sculpted with images of Buddha or deities, or if experienced practiceers especially enchant them, they can be used as highly powerful talismans or amulets.

It is also believed to shield you from ghosts by wearing such amulets or talismans. Also, some think that some stones (White Quartz, Amethyst, Ametrine, Citrine and Smoky Quartz) can offer the same protection, in particular the quartz family. Diamond, pyrite, hamatitis, observian, black star saphire, black diopside, and jet also form other protective stones. I understand myself that the stones have a different degree of electro-magnetic radiation. When worn on our bodies, they serve to strengthen our pulse of body energy, which casts a protective shield over us.

The photo of the Earth Store Bodhisattva made of tektite is a very strong talisman I have. I also have a pyrite and amber necklace, and I use it to be with me while I travel abroad. I have bracelets and pendants made of iron meteorite in my arsenal and they are also very effective in stopping negativity. It is also thought that these moonstones are great defensive stones for travels through waters in general. I still carry in my luggage several bits of tumbled moonstones.

For those afraid of ghosts when they travel abroad and stay in hotel rooms, they can try to put their shoes at the foot of their beds, one with their sole facing up while the other is in the normal position.

Amulets and talismans are also charged by their creators-monks and priests alike-with strong vibrations and serve the same goal as stones. At my point, I can magnetize stones and any objects to give them more radiation by using my energy system or by singing mantras.

Spirits In Rocks, there is belief that some rocks hold memories of the past and some are created to survive for a certain form of life, just as the ermitage crabs, who live on the shell after the shellfish died. Stella my spiritual friend can communicate with stones and said she often saw amazing creatures in some rocks. I once meditated with a labradorite ball (a kind of felspar, transparent with luminous blue and gray background) and the pictures of a woman dressed in the Greek gown in some Roman columns inside the stone. She had ears and forms in almond and was angry with my unwelcome intrusion. There was another rock, a Rhodonite fragment, a pink Manganese steak colored stone, which I could see images in the framework of the dome shape. I recalled another instance when an old lady handed me a jade piece, which she recuperated from her mother's exhumed grave, and asked me if it was okay to wear her lady's daughter. When I picked up my shoes, I felt a painful feeling in my stomach. I asked her if she could remember that her mother had some sort of stomach ailment, and she believed it. I cleansed the stone for her, but she told me she changed her mind and chose to keep it in a jewelry-box instead. Jade is said to have the exceptional value of its owner's security. Whenever the wearer encounters dangerous situations, the legend has it that it covers the hazards on its behalf.

Rocks To draw Chinese luck claims it would be a good fortune to wear such rocks. Jade is the most favored stone adorned not only to give the wearer good luck but also to protect him. For those players who are always hopeful, they should wear yellow precious gemstones-saphir, topaz, or citrines. Some may even carry a pyrite doughnut in their wallet with a dollar coin. Green stones are used to draw career wealth, and not only Jade, but also Emerald, Peridot, Chloride-inclusive Quartz, Aventurine, malachite and Amazonite are part of them. In addition to being used in the rings and pendants as semi-precious stones, some of the stumbling stones—aventurine, malachite, and Amazonite—can be placed on cash registers to maximize day-to-day business takeoffs.

Stones and Feng-shui Feng-Shui and geomancy is also spoken about power-energy from the atmosphere, gravitational forces and currents, seasonal variations in energy flows, celestial and planetary effects, and static object positioning in the world and forms in which your body energy is dealing with and resonating with all these energy sources. Feng-Shui's west application is to locate a range of scientific equipment and to check the different forms of energy in the region. If you are energy-sensitive, then you can feel the influence of "Feng-Shui," the good and evil "Chi" instead of relying entirely on Master's Feng Shui principles. As stones have a positive vibrational power, they can be used to improve the building's feng-shui if it is in the right position. For example, a wealth location is considered to be the left corner of the main hall of the house diagonally opposite the entrance, where one could place amethyst geodes to boost positive energy. This is a better substitute for round leaf plants, as the Feng-shui masters traditionally recommend. We might hang faceted cut crystal balls other than putting mirrors or windscreens at our windows to block negative energy from some of the ill-fashioned structures or landscape facing our house. These faceted balls against sunlight can project spots of rainbow lights into the home and produce a wonderful view as they dance on the walls.

Chapter 6: How Can I Use Crystals To Reduce Stress From Work?

With the use of healing crystals, you can manage everyday stresses effectively while minimizing their effects on your physical, emotional, and spiritual wellbeing. Making use of stress-relieving healing stones in the workplace will ensure that you achieve maximum productivity. It will also help prevent your inner turmoils from affecting your relationship with your co-workers and your clients.

Recommended Crystals for the Workplace

Amber

Amber stones are effective in providing you with the necessary courage for establishing relationship boundaries. So if you're the type of person who's not very good in maintaining employer-employee borders or if you're having issues with your relations with clients, then consider owning this gemstone.

Emerald

This gemstone symbolizes abundance. Use this to achieve mental clarity while visualizing wealth and prosperity.

Amethyst

When you find it particularly challenging to control a current work situation or when you would like to alter unwanted realities in your workplace, then an amethyst can serve as a valuable ally.

Purple Fluorite

Place a cluster of these stones right next to the computer to shield you from the negative effects of its electromagnetic field.

Garnet

If you feel like the energy levels in the office are a bit low, a garnet can help boost that overall energy.

Blue Lace Agate

If you find it difficult to communicate with co-workers, clients, or persons of authority, the Blue Lace Agate can help you improve your communication skills. Furthermore, it will provide you with courage to speak the truth. Use this stone when you feel like you're voice is often unheard and misunderstood.

Bloodstone

This gemstone is perfect for individuals seeking more motivation. Running out of brilliant ideas lately? This crystal will help enhance your creativity.

Smoky Quartz

The workplace can be filled with emotional vampires, from your toxic co-worker to your verbally abusive boss. Use this gemstone to protect yourself from this draining of energy. This gem will assist you in being more emotionally secure and shield you from self-doubt.

Citrine

The Success Stone is helpful in improving your problem-solving skills.

Larimar

This is the ideal crystal to be used for opening communication pathways within the workplace. Use this when you're having difficulty listening to and understanding others around you.

Rainbow Obsidian

Been forgetful lately? This gemstone is recommended if you wish to improve your memory. It will prevent you from missing important meetings and skipping important stuff in your to-do list.

How do I use these crystals?

You can harness the energy and the stress-fighting effects of these crystals in the workplace in many ways. As previously discussed, you may carry the stones in your pocket or fasten them inside your clothes. Alternatively, you may use them as worry stones.

Another way is by placing the stones on your desk or in a sacred place in your workstation where they will be visible to you most of the time. Every time you look at these healing rocks, they will serve as a constant reminder for you to achieve mindfulness in everything that you do.

One more method is by creating a healing crystal grid in your workspace or in your home.

How to Make a Crystal Grid

While healing crystals are powerful on their own, crystal grids are able to combine all the energies of multiple healing stones as well as their scared geometries with the power of your intentions. As such, this yields quicker, more effective results.

The primary step in creating a crystal grid is to identify your intention. Is your goal to invite wealth and abundance? Do you want to maintain your health goals and to reduce stress? Do you want to be able to sleep better at night? The crystals that you will choose to include in your grid will depend greatly on your goal. For instance, crystal grids dedicated for the purpose of health and wellness should make use of mostly blue and purple crystals like Fluorite and Sodalite. Alternatively, you may trust your instincts and select stones that speak to you. You'll notice that when you purchase crystals from a store, certain crystals' energies communicate more strongly to you than others'.

In order to create your healing crystal grid, you need to select a location in your home or in your workspace. Make sure that it is somewhere where the grid won't be disturbed.

Then write down your intention on a piece of paper. The more specific it is, the better.

Clear the energy of the room by burning some sage or by placing a bowl of sea salt in the room. This is to make the space suitable for your grid.

Then, place the piece of paper with your intention right in the middle of the crystal grid cloth.

Afterwards, take a deep breath and speak out your intention. Alternatively, you may choose to envision your goal in your mind's eye.

There should be a center crystal that is placed right in the middle of the cloth. To arrange the surrounding crystals, start from the outside moving towards the center. With each crystal that you place, make sure that you are thinking of your intention. Then, place the center crystal on top of the piece of paper.

The next thing to do would be to activate the crystal grid. This is done by using a quartz crystal point. Beginning from the outside, you should trace an invisible line between each of the crystals to link each stone with the one beside it.

Finally, you may choose to add candles to enhance the effect of your crystal grid. Allow it the grid to stay in place for at least forty days.

Chapter 7: Tips For Selecting Healing Crystals

For a better balance of your physical, mental, spiritual, and emotional health you can make use of the stones, crystals, and other Earth elements. Do not think of this practice as a replacement for required healthcare, instead use crystal healing as a complementary practice. Those of you who are suffering from serious problems related to health should consult your doctor or healthcare provider.

Tip 1: Feel the energy emanating from the stone

While you are selecting healing stones, it is essential that you hold this stone in your hand and try feeling how the energy emanating from the stone is interacting with your own energy. The next step is that you should close your eyes and see if you can feel any slight sensations such as tingling in either your hands or arms.

While doing this also pay close attention to any sensations in other parts of your body that might get affected because of the energy from the stones. Further, pay close attention to any other sensations or emotions that are produced because of the stone. For those who cannot touch and experience their crystals before making the purchase, for instance if you are ordering crystals online, there is one simple thing you can do. Go to a quiet place and close your eyes. After you have closed your eyes, focus on the stone and see how the stone makes you feel on a physical, emotional, mental, and spiritual level.

Tip 2: Clean the Stones

If you want your crystals to maintain their vibrations over time, you will need to cleanse your crystals. Even after making a new purchase of crystals you should cleanse them thoroughly before putting them to use and also cleanse them every few days when they are used. Two of the easiest ways to cleanse your crystals is by either placing them in the sunlight or the moonlight for a couple of hours. If the stone is capable of getting wet, then even running it under tap water also helps. Other suggestions for cleansing your crystals are mentioned in detail in the coming chapters.

Tip 3: Program your Stones

Intention plays a critical role while you are making use of stones, crystals, or any other Earth elements for the purpose of physical and energy healing. After you have cleansed the stones or crystals, you will have to program them with your intention. Programming the stone is quite simple, all that you have to do is place these stones in your hands and meditate with them. While you are meditating, you will have to transfer the energy of intention to the stone. For instance, let us assume that you want to cleanse you aura. The stone you will use for this purpose is quartz; while meditating you will have to imagine this stone cleansing the aura and make an affirmative statement signifying that the stone will be used in this way.

Tip 4: Research

It is quintessential that you do some research for gathering information about not just the healing properties of the stone but also the ways to use them. You can do so by either looking up the information available in a reliable website or even gather knowledge by reading a book related to this topic.

Tip 5: Ways to work with the stones

Different users work with healing stones in different ways. It is not necessary that everyone use them in the same fashion. You can hold the stones in your hands while meditating or while praying. You can also incorporate these healing crystals into your jewelry. Similarly, when you are trying to align your chakras, you can place these stones on or near the chakras so that you can balance your energies.

Chapter 8: Choosing Healing Crystals For Anxiety And Stress

The scope of precious stones that can be utilized for recuperating is colossal; however, with regards to conditions, for example, nervousness and worry, some are more favored than others so if you are looking for stones to assist you with these conditions, you should need to look at a portion of the ones underneath.

Amethyst is A Master Healer

Amethyst is one of the precious stones that are known to have the option to help with a wide assortment of conditions. For tension issues and loosening up, this is one of the most well known. This is known to be the Master Healer, and it has a quieting impact on the body and psyche, in addition to it is one of the better looking precious stones for putting around the home.

Sea green/blue the Calming Stone

Sea green/blue is a beautiful looking gem that can help with issues identified with nervousness and fits of anxiety. This is notable for having the option to assist the individual with relaxing and quiet alongside calming the brain. Sea green/blue is known for its properties of bringing down the degrees of stress.

Clear Quartz Dispels Negativity

Clear Quartz precious stone might probably help individuals to oversee tension as it has properties of scattering negative speculation alongside transforming negative musings into increasingly positive contemplations. This is one of the manifestations that individuals often grumble about when enduring fits of anxiety.

Moonstone Calms Panic

Fits of anxiety can devastatingly affect the life of an individual, and one of the precious stones that numerous individuals partner with them is Moonstone. This stone stops over response to circumstances; thus, it is often the decision of the individuals who use precious stones for recuperating frenzy and tension.

Smokey Quartz Alleviates Stress

Smokey Quartz is often utilized by individuals who use recuperating precious stones as it is known for its properties identified with having the option to calm pressure that is related to uneasiness.

Utilizing Your Crystals

There are numerous ways that you can utilize any of the above gems for facilitating nervousness and making your life less unpleasant. Natural approaches incorporate reflection and lighting a flame and enabling it to glimmer on your preferred gemstone. You can utilize them for holding in the palm to decrease feelings of anxiety, or you should need to lay down with them under your pad to help cut down the degrees of stress and nervousness.

There truly isn't any single direction that works when utilizing gems for recuperating, so you should need to give different ways before settling a shot, the one that is directly for you.

Crystal Energy Healing and Its Many Benefits

Crystal Energy Healing for Mind, Body, and Spirit is cultivated by bringing into parity four major regions of the body.

CHAKRA BALANCE: Balancing the chakras permits legitimate vitality stream to the cells and expanding vitality in your body. You utilize a similar essential procedure for every one of the seven Chakra regions.

Mind BALANCE: Brain equalization is for putting your privilege and left cerebrum halves of the globe again into parity. On an everyday premise, the more significant part of us utilizes one side of the mind more than the other. Given the tremendous measures of pressure and tension we each face, these halves of the globe of the brain are regularly out of parity.

CIRCULATORY BALANCE: The circulatory framework is the water-powered procedure of development of liquids in the body. By adjusting the circulatory arrangement of the body, the body can all the more effectively transport oxygen through the blood and divert poisons. This makes a far healthier internal environment prompting slower aging.

NEUROLOGICAL BALANCE: adjusts the meridians, the attractive internal streamlines of the body. At the point when the extremities of the body are in equalization, there are fewer vitality blockages. You will encounter a sentiment of restored vitality, and the body can all the more effectively convey recuperating energy to where it is required.

Dissimilar to numerous types of vitality mending, Crystal Energy Healing does not require months or long stretches of study. You can figure out how to utilize crystals for mending the Mind, Body, and Spirit in only a couple of short sessions. The majority of what you have to know can be aced inside an hour, and from that point on, it is extremely a matter of building up your intuitive stream.

Before you start you will need to have, 2 Crystal for yourself, 2 Crystals for the Client and a seat or a spot for the customer to set down.

You will likewise need to learn Techniques to shield yourself and your customer from outside energies and the exchanges of energies from yourself to the customer or visa Versa.

Just as utilizing crystals for the adjusting of Mind, Body, and Spirit as referenced above, you can likewise use your glasses to do Aura Scanning, Relieve torment and strain.

As should be obvious, the advantages of Crystal Energy Healing are numerous and changed. There isn't sufficient room in an individual section to go into the systems for each progression.

Aura Alignment With Crystal Energy

Aura arrangement is something that isn't encouraged much in vitality work, yet it is a specific piece of understanding and working inside your aura fields. Presently we as a whole have seven noteworthy aura layers/handle that we exist in, and each layer compares to the other issue inside our life. Aura arrangement is actually what it says it is, adjusting the auras!

Think about our auras as like huge air pockets that encompass us. One is slightly higher than the other one, enveloping the previous aura layer and the majority of its issues. Presently when you are getting an image in your mind, high since that is the thing that we need. Currently, envision that one of those air pockets move slightly askew. What will occur? Typically, when they were useful air pockets, they would pop. What happens when your aura layers are not adjusted is that they begin finding each other making lively flotsam and jetsam free, and this would then be able to cloud your aura or cause stale vitality. Presently in light of the fact that you find stale energy or an obfuscated atmosphere on someone, or yourself, does not always mean they have a misadjusted aura - as you as the practitioner need to explore the vitality issues close by and find the underlying cause, as recall that we as a whole have distinctive vitality marks that we reverberate inside.

So what would you be able to do to re-adjust your aura? Gem mending utilizing Citrine works best for this! Make sure to ground and focus yourself before you start an aura arrangement session. Get one bit of Citrine in each hand, and make enormous clearing movements over your aura field, turning yourself clockwise in action. Do this for in any event 5 minutes and after that rests on your back and place one bit of Citrine on each side at your palm chakras for an additional 10 minutes. This will enable the energies to be retained and re-adjust your aura layers. Ensure you purify your gems after every session you perform!

Crystal For Healing

Are Precious stones pretty shakes, right? They come in every unique shading pinks, blues, greens; and they make for incredible paperweights, yet what can that dusty hunk of shake you once purchased spontaneously from a store that smelt excessively firmly of incense accomplish for you? Well for one, you can utilize a gem for mending.

Precious stones, similar to Aladdin's light, are more than what they appear. Their shrouded perspectives have been cut in the rock by old Egyptians and written in the material by the Babylonians. Indeed, even today, the windows of Tiffany's and Cartier are a demonstration of our fixation on precious stones and gemstones. Maybe the reason we prize them has more to do with how they affect us than we might suspect.

Any evident researcher will reveal to you that all gems have energy or charge that isn't so not the same as the human body. So envision what you can do with this free energy! Studies demonstrate that when put in water, it changes the sub-atomic structure of the fluid, it transmits vibrations, and innovation can even take photographs of a precious stones energy field. So as opposed to utilizing gems to transduce and transmit energy in PCs, TV's, and looks as they are being used, today-you can use them to recuperate, adjust, quiet, and make.

At the point when the energy body, air or chakras of you or I, is aggravated or out of parity, it directly affects our physical body- muscle hurts, skin inflammation, joint inflammation, and so on! A gems singular properties can be utilized to work in agreement with the human body to transmute or even intensify certain angles in your energy body using three straightforward advances:

1. Picking your gem

Gems are not any different, and when picking one for a particular reason, it is educated. Like jewels, cut, shading, clarity, and size all have any effect. In any case, remember, a crude and shady precious stone has as much power as a cleaned one, just in various ways. Complete a bit of perusing and find what you are searching for. When you feel a little overpowered, remember the intensity of instinct!!

2. Purifying and charging your precious stone

There are various approaches to purify your gem so it is cleared of any past vibrations or negative energies and it's to you to choose which one you feel is ideal. My preferred strategy is to put the precious stone in a bowl of water and leave it outside during a waxing moon night. Another popular route is to put it in a bunch of amethyst or clear quartz precious stones for 12 hours. Keep in mind that your precious stone is always absorbing outside energy, so it requires frequent purifying for ideal use.

3. Becoming more acquainted with your precious stone

Your precious stone can complete a ton for you yet you have to discover its quality and why this stone was shaped in the earth miles from your doorstep has come into your life. Without a doubt, you went out and got it-however it has a specific vibration and energy that is exceptional, much the same as you. Become acquainted with its energy stream and your recuperating will work much better.

For:

Certainty: Carry or think with Green jasper. This stone invigorates the blood course and the heart chakra giving quality and endurance.

Rejuvenation: Red garnet is an incredibly refreshing stone. Spot a garnet in a glass of water for a moment and after that drink to kick you begin to your day!

Unwinding: An extraordinary strategy to accomplish general mending is by putting eight amethyst gems around you when resting. These precious stones, quiet feelings, and help reflection and rest. Attempt distinctive layout patterns to balances what works best for you.

So residue off your crystalline paperweight and have a ton of fun with your precious stones place them in your water, convey them in your pocket, and maybe the

Crystal Age of Atlantis won't feel like such a legend all things considered.

How to Use Chakra Crystals

The main principle behind chakra treatment is that there are seven energy focuses on different focuses on the body. It is said that putting the right stones on these focuses of energy can help in the recuperating procedure. There is nobody stone that works for everybody or even on each energy focus. You may need to test yet by recognizing what works for other people, and you may locate a beginning stage for yourself.

It is said that the human body is encompassed by energy and that by setting gems on the body at specific focuses, you can change the progression of power. This positive energy would then be able to calm pressure and advance characteristic mending. This is much equivalent to helping your body to mend with herbs and minerals.

Most use either a solitary precious stone or a little strand of gems. These ought to be in regular structure with no metals encompassing them for the best impact. The shade of the precious stone just as the quality can significantly affect how well it functions and in which territories.

It is frequently prescribed that these be utilized as a deterrent medication instead of for mending. The energy from the gems might be used to improve the progression of power from your body and help in keeping negative energy from causing ailment and physical diseases.

You ought to comprehend that these may not work for every individual, and the impacts might be diverse for every person. For the ideal outcomes, you might need to counsel somebody who thinks about the properties of each stone and how best to utilize them to accomplish the results you are looking for.

Chakra precious stones can be incredible for those trying to expel negative energy or improve the nature of power their body is utilizing. These may likewise be useful in enhancing the measure of strength your body has to use every day. Indeed, even the most doubtful scientists concur that the human body needs energy to mend and capacity. Why not check whether chakra treatment can help reestablish your parity of positive energy today?

Uses of Crystals

These days, Crystals are found in the market in a wide range of shapes, sizes, and hues. For the most part, individuals are befuddled, considering which kind of precious stones they ought to utilize. A large number of them give the least consideration to which stone they should purchase. They don't make sure if the stone is perfect with their zodiac signs. It is continuously viewed as better if the individual zodiac signs pick the precious stones. Along these lines, it will be helpful to your wellbeing and you, as choosing an off-base precious stone may influence your wellbeing as well as affect your social and expert life.

There are a wide range of uses of these precious stones, for example,

1. Utilized for mending: It is accepted that precious stones help fix ailments and agonies in the body. Likewise, it professes to decontaminate your body and increment your energy levels. It also claims to decontaminate your quality. In this procedure, the air's layers are purified. There are seven layers which must be cleaned and recuperated. This is currently utilized as one of the methods for sedating an individual.

2. Utilized for reflection: Meditation is being done since days of yore. Also, presently, the holy people accept that by using gems into consideration, your enthusiasm is quieted down. You don't

wind up being hyperactive. Likewise, it is said that your soul is lifted.

3. Utilized for feng shui: It is accepted that precious stones assume an outstanding job in improving the feng shui of a house. It is said that by keeping precious stones in the house, sound energy is kept up. What's more, the right energy circling in a home is always valuable.

4. Utilized for pendulums: Pendulums are being used for numerous years. With the utilization of a precious stone in a swing, the excellence of the artistry additionally improves, and the pendulums are felt perfect and extraordinary given their properties.

5. Utilized for adjusting of chakras: "Chakras" are those spots of the body which help to make our collection unadulterated. They are viewed as energy focuses of the body. There are seven places in our body. Along these lines, our body is made free from illnesses and

torments. The precious stones are put on these "chakras" for mending the piece of the body. The precious stones are placed on various chakras relying upon how the adjusting is to be finished.

6. Utilized for making glass: Crystal is lovely to take a gander at. In this way, it is used to create an extraordinary sort of drink. It gives a beautiful look.

These were the significant uses of gems.

Crystal Healing Therapy

Chakra Balancing and Crystal Healing

Gems in recuperating are performed with gemstones and pearls which are situated on the body in different, explicit zones. These regions are called chakras. You will discover seven noteworthy chakras with a lot increasingly minor ones that are utilized during the time spent precious stone mending. These optional chakras are known as meridians. Chakras are various focuses on the body that precious stones are put on to have the option to achieve or create specific outcomes.

Merely alluding to the chakras alone is undoubtedly an in-depth, intriguing exchange. What every means and exactly how every one of them meets up on the planet of gem mending is positively not shy of stunning. Each chakra has its shading and possesses "work" to keep the psyche, body, and soul joined together and cooperating as opposed to getting to be uneven. The act of precious stone recuperating has existed for quite a long time and has just gotten progressively notable as the years have cruised by. It had been initially used in Eastern societies with utilizations, for example, shielding from shrewdness spirits and adversity, however, has been advancing West, that it is presently no longer an unexpected when individuals notice precious stone recuperating as a method for bringing the brain, body, and soul into the arrangement.

There is no logical evidence that gem mending works, yet when you experience the declarations of those who've profited in significant ways from this, there is unquestionably some legitimacy to it that doesn't begin from having the option to be demonstrated through science. As everybody knows, numerous things can't be shown through science, yet it doesn't make it any less genuine or any less substantial.

In contrast to conventional medication, precious stone mending takes a shot at the entire individual, personality, body, and soul, and doesn't merely focus on the physical perspective that requires recuperating. It has been said that utilizing precious stones can anticipate disease in an individual's life. It isn't terrible for do, as long as the individual using the gems doesn't disregard individual security and wellbeing. Investigate gem recuperating weight reduction of an inseparable arrangement with a drug when it's required, rather than a swap for customary therapeutic practices.

Among the easiest ways that individuals have joined precious stone treatment into their lives is to put gems around their homes and work environments and even on themselves. Guarantee that you put recuperating precious stones inside a spot that you could see and that is secured against daylight alongside other harm. They might be acclimated with make specific kinds of vitality or states of mind, to make unwinding, and furthermore to wash down nature. Precious stones produce a domain of harmony and warmth and mending that can penetrate each factor of your lifetime. They are well worth exploring to perceive how they can carry stunning changes to any or all that you do.

The Top Five Crystals For Developing Your Psychic Abilities

Many precious stones can be utilized to help with clairvoyant improvement. However, some have different characteristics which are a reward and will likewise urge you to, in addition to other things, work correctly, convey better, build up your natural blessings thus considerably more. This best five are magnificent stones to work with, particularly for fledglings.

Amethyst is anything but difficult to discover and one of the most widely recognized gems for mystic improvement. Its hues run from pale lavender through to profound purple and can without much of a stretch be found as groups, tumblestones, decorations, and gems. Amethyst has a high spiritual vibration and a defensive quality-a right blend for clairvoyant advancement work. Amethyst encourages profound contemplation and more top conditions of mindfulness. It additionally assists with mental control and center, opening your instinct, and increasing spiritual understanding and intelligence. Amethyst enacts the third eye chakra, which is in charge of may parts of clairvoyant advancement.

Clear Quartz is exceptionally simple to lay your hands on and sensibly valued. It intensifies vitality, which is one of the principal reasons it is one of the most exceedingly prescribed precious stones for clairvoyant work. Am I not catching this' meaning? Indeed, when you need to build your capacity to 'hear,' 'see ' or' know' messages from your instinct, mystic side, our soul guides, you have to consider yourself a beneficiary, much like a pole or satellite dish. The words are coming to you. However, you may not be fixed on them, or can't hear them. Clear quartz can intensify their vitality, making them 'more intense' and all the more clear for you. Clear quartz additionally adjusts you to your spiritual purpose.

Celestite is light blue and sparkly. It is a genuinely peaceful stone, associated with the other-worldly domains. It has an amicable vitality, quieting and honing the brain. It is extraordinary for amateurs or the individuals who have not done any mystic improvement work for some time as it can kick off your capacities and animate unique insight. It shows trust and confidence in the celestial, or the master plan - that everything has meant so creates comprehension and tolerance on your clairvoyant improvement venture.

Sodalite is a mottled mid to dull blue with white veins. It has a delicate vitality that causes you to keep a coherent personality while additionally promising your instinct and spiritual discernment - a fantastic mix when working mystically. Sodalite extends reflection and animates the third eye chakra. It is an excellent stone for a clairvoyant advancement gathering or hovers as it improves trust, friendship, and concordance. Moreover, blue is the shade of correspondence, so it bodes well to utilize while attempting to empower telepathic communication.

Tigers Eye is usually a dull darker and yellow-gold stripey stone that when cleaned to a tumblestone consistently helps me to remember a sham. There are red and blue tigers eye precious stones, and they have other properties. Like amethyst, tigers eye invigorated the third eye chakra yet, also, has defensive characteristics. It brings out honesty - essential when passing messages to others in your mystic advancement work, and encourages you to perceive your gifts, capacities, and furthermore shortcomings or defects (so you can enhance them).

Try not to feel you have to convey these stones to help you in your work, and one will do pleasantly. Or on the other hand, you could substitute them and see which works best for you. You may locate that one assist with one component of your work, while another encourages an alternate angle or aptitude.

Using Crystals For Healing

The utilization of precious stones for mending goes back to the old Greeks and Indians who accepted there were huge pearls that offered light to a different universe under their known world. So utilizing gems for recuperating today isn't generally such new, It is still exceptionally successful and significantly increasingly refined today.

We can discover precious stones around us regular and continuously, they are in our watches, PCs, PDAs, etc. Precious stones, stones, and shakes are living thick substances that emit energy and can adjust zones of our bodies and atmosphere. The use of stones or gems inside explicit energy centers (chakras) draws light and shading into the body's emanation and with this light can empower recuperating.

Precious stones are thought to center or generally change energy to invigorate mending. They can be utilized for recuperating, and there is an extraordinary nature joined to gems. Explicit precious stones are proposed to treat a wide assortment of physical and passionate conditions including bursitis, cerebral pains, acid reflux, sleep deprivation, hemorrhages, ailment, thrombosis, absent-mindedness, nervousness, sadness, Parkinson's sickness, visual deficiency, and disease.

All gems have their very own quality and are lovely. You can convey precious stones in your pocket, wear them on a chain, place them in shower water, or spot them in your home to bring the intensity of mending inside reach. Various sorts and shades of stones or precious stones are elevated to have diverse mending forces and a few people guarantee certain gemstones or gems convey exceptional energy that can be moved to individuals to give insurance against infection, reestablish wellbeing, and provide otherworldly direction.

There are bunches of incredible uses for precious stones, you can set a gem in your pets water bowl to keep water unadulterated, new and gainful or you can put a flower in your feline's water bowl for cleansing and spot gems on your felines bed, underpads, on tabletops spot gems around the house for congruity grasp one while stroking your felines or simply unwinding for mystic work, energy mending, and generally speaking health. When a month you should put your gems in the sun to energize them, other than quartz, as they can get so hot that they can begin a flame.

Individuals who practice different recuperating expressions regularly like their gems somewhat shady for establishing themselves or the patient. A few healers like gems with a ton of character and characteristics in their appearance, likewise they like them to be crude and unpolished. At the point when treasures are uncovered, it is said they have increasingly female energy, called yin so if the healer is dealing with recuperating ladylike energy, they will utilize a gem from the earth.

Chapter 9: Crystal Care

Crystals are beautiful elements that vibrate with energy and have the power to transform your life positively. When you get yourself a crystal, you are not just an owner of the gemstone but also its guardian. Crystals speak to us in myriad ways, and therefore, it is important to care for them and ensure that their channels of communication remain open and clear.

Crystals are direct gifts to humankind given to us by Mother Earth, and it is our duty to guard their powers and make sure they do not lose their shine as well as their capabilities to improve our lives. Considering the importance of looking after crystals well in order to have access to their limitless powers. It makes sense to dedicate a chapter to the care of crystals. So, here goes.

When to Cleanse Crystals

All newly bought or received crystals have to be cleansed before you use them. After the first time of cleansing is over, the next time you need to do it, you will know. As the crystals accumulate negative energies, they lose their original luster and characteristic traits, which will give you an indication that it is time to cleanse your gemstone.

For example, clear quartz will become cloudier than usual instead of being clear and transparent. Some crystals, in fact, become heavy and dense when they have gathered excessive negative energies. Also, the frequency of cleansing and recharging your crystals depend on their usage.

If you use them regularly like wearing them on your body as pieces of jewelry or keep them in your home to keep your home free of negative energy, then you will have to cleanse them more often than if you use a big crystal occasionally for healing purposes. Most importantly, you will not get optimum output from your crystals when they are in dire need of cleansing and recharging.

Additionally, if you want to reprogram your crystal with a different intention, then you must clear it off the earlier intention.

Cleansing and Charging Crystals

The primary purpose of cleansing crystals to purify and honor them. It is a sacred process, which helps you pay gratitude to the stone as well as the universe for nurturing the crystal and making it ready for your use. The cleansing ritual also includes giving thanks to Mother Earth for transferring her powers into the stone.

Moreover, by the time crystals reach you, they are likely to have absorbed different kinds of energy into their bosoms including the negative and harmful ones. As you use crystals too, they continue to absorb these energies from their surroundings. Therefore, regular cleansing of crystals that takes care of clearing accumulate negative energies should be undertaken without fail. There are many ways of cleansing your crystals. Let us look at some of them.

Soaking in salt water - Take some alkaline water in a glass bowl and add ½ teaspoon of sea salt for every cup. Stir the salt in the water until it is completely dissolved. Put your crystal in this water making sure the stone is entirely submerged. Now, close your eyes and hover your palms over the submerged crystal.

Set the intention for the negative energies of the crystals to be removed. Let the crystals soak in the bowl of water overnight. Remove it in the morning and rinse it thoroughly ensuring the edges, if any, do not have any crystals of salt stuck in them. Salt water is a great cleanser for crystals like aquamarine, Iolite, Sodalite, Blue Lace Agate, Blue Quartz, etc.

Rinsing them under running water - If you have access to a water spring or water fountain, then placing them under this running water is a great way to cleanse and charge your crystals. However, some crystals should not be cleansed using plain water or salt water because they have a tendency to break or get damaged.

Smudging - Hold the crystals in your hand or place them in a bowl. Light a small bundle of sage until it smolders and smoke begins to emit out. Wave this smoke over the crystal. After you feel the negative energies have all gone from your crystal, you can put out the embers.

While the most potent element for effective smudging is white sage, you can also use Palo Santo wood or sweet grass. It is best to use a fire-proof glass or ceramic bowl to hold your crystal for smudging.

Using the power of sound - For this, you need something called a singing bowl, which rings at a particular frequency when it is struck. Place the crystal you want to be cleansed close to the singing bowl, and strike the bowl thrice. Now, hold the crystal and guide it over the rim of the bowl so that the sound waves are caught by the stone. If the crystals are small enough to fit into the singing bowl, then place them inside, and then strike the bowl for the sound. The sound waves help in eliminating negative energies accumulated in the crystal.

Using white light - White light also referred to as universal light is a powerful cleanser of crystals. Anyone can create this white light. Close your eyes and speak to your divine spirit or any other god or goddess you believe in, and ask him or her to create white light for you. This approach works like a powerful prayer.

Now, imagine your entire body filled with this pure, white light. Open your eyes and using small sweeping hand gestures direct the white light to the crystal that needs to be cleansed. Ask the divine power you believe in to clear the negative energies accumulated in the crystal.

Using Tibetan chimes - Also called Tingsha hand cymbals, these instruments are fairly light and small to carry around. Resonating with a high vibration, these chimes have the power to clear negative energies from everywhere including crystals. Just move them around and touch them together to produce a high-pitched sound, which can clear disharmony in the surroundings as well as eliminate all negative energies from the crystals in the vicinity.

Using rice - Brown or white rice is great for crystal cleansing. Rice is great for crystals, which cannot be cleansed using water, or by smudging. Take some rice in a ceramic bowl and place the crystals over it. Leave this arrangement overnight. The rice will simply absorb all the negative energies from the crystals. Remember to throw away the rice and not use it in your cooking.

Using a quartz cluster - Some crystals are great for cleansing purposes. For example, a cluster of citrine or clear quartz can be used for this purpose. This arrangement is great for small pieces of crystals such as those embedded in rings and earrings. Place these pieces of jewelry on the cluster and leave them there overnight. Remember to use a soft piece of cloth to prevent scratches and other damage to both your crystal cluster as well as the small stone that is being cleansed.

Burying your crystals - It is possible to clear negative powers accumulated in your crystals by burying them in earth. Simply bury your crystals in a safe spot and mark it so that you can recover your stones when they are cleansed and ready.

Placing them in sunlight or moonlight - Place your crystals in a ceramic bowl and leave them in a spot that gets the direct moonlight on a full-moon night or from a crescent moon. Leave them like this at least for 7-10 hours. This process will clear crystals of negative energy and fill them with positive energy so that stones are charged up to do your bidding.

Programming Crystals

Programming your crystal is way of transferring your intention to it so that it can help you achieve certain objectives and desires. Here are some steps you can follow to program your crystals with any specific intention.

• First, determine the objective or desire you want to achieve. Then, choose the crystal for this specific purpose. Ask the crystal if it is willing to partner with you in achieving your goal.

• You will find a powerfully strong resistance is the crystal's intentions are not aligned with your purpose. As you practice crystal healing, you will notice that determining a no is very easy because you will feel a strong resistance. A yes could simply get a neutral response.

- Next, hold the crystal close to your heart chakra, and then to your third eye chakra. As you do this, repeat your intention in your mind or even mouth your intentions softly. Visualize the task being projected into the crystal as you hold the stone close to your body.

- Hold the stone in your hand in front of you until the crystal, heart chakra, and the third eye chakra connect with each other in the form of triangle.

- Say your intention out loud and hold this position until you feel satisfied that the crystals is charged with the task.

- Finally, thank the crystal for participating in your endeavor and for being a willing partner to help you.

Storing Your Crystals

Storing your crystals when not in use is as important as cleansing and charging them regularly. Here are some pointers regarding how to store your gemstones:

Choose a dry and clean place to store them. Crystals can be damaged if they are exposed to salty and moisture-laden environments like coastal areas. Also, make sure there is no dust in and around the place you are storing your crystals.

It makes sense to invest in a nice box covered in velvet cloth to keep your special pieces. Boxes made of good quality plastic or non-corrosive materials are best suited for this.

Using these kinds of safe materials ensures there is no chemical reaction with the stone. Covered boxes protect crystals and keep them safe from the vagaries of external environments.

Avoid using cotton pads to hold the crystals because the edges of your special stones could catch the fibers, which could get stuck there. However, you can use cotton pads as a soft holder for tumbled stones. In fact, you can keep any polished stone in most of the common places from where you can access it. For example, you can keep them in your pocket, on your desk, under your pillow while sleeping, in water (of course after making sure that the stone has no poisonous attributes), or anywhere else. Physical

Small, soft, and fragile pieces are best kept in separate holders because physical brushing with other crystals could damage them. A great way to store small pieces of jewelry is to use egg holders typically used to store eggs in refrigerators.

FAQs for Crystal Care

Here are some frequently asked questions to give you a nice summary of crystal care along with some value-added information too:

How frequently should I clean my crystals?

The more frequently you use your crystals, the more negative energy they will gather, and therefore, will need to be cleaned often. If you think a particular crystal seems heavier than normal, then this too is an indication that it needs to be cleaned. There are no hard and fast rules to clean your crystals though you can go by the thumb rule that all crystals need to be cleaned and recharged at least once a month.

What is the sign that the crystal has been cleansed well?

After a crystal is cleansed well, you will find it lighter than before and also be able to feel and connect to its psychic energy much more easily than before. The denseness will have reduced and, in some cases, the crystals will shed the cloudiness and regain their original clarity and transparency.

Which is the best cleansing and charging method?

There is no one solution-fits-all answer for this question. Every crystal is unique and has different characteristic properties. Moreover, cleansing methods also are specific to an individual. What works for someone else may not work for you because your own energy vibrations are different and unique. Therefore, try all the methods mentioned in this chapter, and choose one or two that works best for you.

Also, some crystals dissolve in water. For such crystals, you must not use plain water, running water, or salt water to clean. Similarly, some crystals could get damaged if you bury them under the earth for cleansing. So, it is imperative that you treat each crystal differently and choose a cleansing method that is best suited for you and for the particular stone.

Chapter 10: Healing With Crystals

Simply owning a few healing crystals and wearing them from time to time isn't going to change your life. Just like with everything else, crystal healing takes some time and a little bit of effort. It isn't much, but you do need to put in some work. But the results are well worth it. There are so many ways in which crystals can improve your life.

Crystals and Chakras

Chakras are a very important part of life, especially when it comes to energy, and so, understanding how chakras work will always be a requirement for proper crystal healing.

What Are Chakras?

Like blood, energy flows throughout the entire body. It travels along set pathways and circulates in a single direction. This energy plays an important role in the health of your mind, body, and spirit. Irregularities in the flow of energy can have severe consequences, and it is important to keep the flow as steady as possible. Throughout the body, there are seven main energy centers throughout the body called chakras. These chakras send your energy throughout the rest of your body and manage the balance and flow of your energy. They act almost like gateways, opening and closing to limit the amount of energy allowed through. The first of the seven chakras is found at the base of the spine and run in a line to the crown of the head. Each chakra has its own function and represents important elements of life. Each chakra also has a color assigned to it that represents its purpose and the type of energy it works with.

The first chakra is called the root chakra, or Muladhara. It sits at the very base of your spine, near your tailbone. The purpose of this chakra is to ground you by connecting all your energy to the earth. It creates stability and is responsible for everything you need to survive from day to day. This chakra is associated with the color red. The most common signs of a balanced root chakra are a sense of accomplishment when thinking about elements such as safety and financial stability, and a strong feeling of being connected to your human experience. An overactive root chakra can cause unease, jitteriness, paranoia, digestive problems, hip pain, and lower back issues. An underactive chakra can sap your concentration and prevent your thoughts from staying grounded in the moment. The most easily recognizable sign is an unhealthy amount of daydreaming.

The second chakra is called the sacral chakra, also known as Svadhishana. This chakra is located just below the belly button and is focused on the self. This chakra is centered around your identity as a human being living on this earth, here and now. It encourages you to enjoy and appreciate the fruits of your hard labor and provides creative energy. The sacral chakra helps you enjoy life and is connected to the color orange. A balanced chakra will help you find more pleasure in the good things in life, but also avoid overdoing them. It will be easier for you to find inspiration in things like good food, intimacy and creative activities and you will feel good about and satisfied by them. An overactive sacral chakra can cause gluttony, obesity, hormone imbalances and addiction. An underactive chakra may lead to impotence, depression, and a devastating lack of creativity and passion.

Third is the solar plexus chakra, or Manipura. It is located at the center of your belly button and is the source of your self-confidence, personal power, and identity as an individual. This is where your "gut-feelings" come from when you instinctively know a person, location, or situation just isn't right for you. The solar plexus chakra is connected to the color yellow and helps you feel empowered, wiser, more decisive and more confident in who you are. It is often called the warrior chakra, as a perfectly balanced chakra creates the same feeling as a warrior going into battle, confident in his ability to win and wise enough to understand what he is fighting for. An overactive solar plexus chakra can lead to a short temper, greed, a lack of empathy and sympathy, and a strong need to micromanage and be in control at all times. It can also lead to issues with your digestive system and severe problems with your internal organs. An underactive solar plexus chakra can cause indecision, insecurity, a lack of energy and a tendency to be needy.

Your heart chakra - or Anahata - is next. It is located in your chest directly over your heart. It deals with strong emotions and especially love for both yourself and others. It is also strongly associated with growth and healing, which is why it is represented by the color green. It can help you see the goodness and compassion in others during tough times and allows you to love and appreciate yourself and other people in equal measures. An overactive heart chakra can cause you to always prioritize the needs of others above your own to an unhealthy extent. It can cause serious problems in your relationship with yourself and often leads to palpitations, an increased heart rate and heartburn. If your heart chakra is underactive, it can close you off from others and prevent you from building deep relationships. You can feel disconnected from your body and suffer from circulation problems as well.

The fifth chakra is the throat chakra, also called Vishuddha. This one sits right in the center of your collarbone and empowers communication and lets you speak your personal truths with clarity and confidence. It is just above your heart chakra and is thus also connected to love and compassion. The throat chakra lets you speak more easily from the heart. It helps you find the right words to carry your message over and to inspire those around you. It is associated with the color blue. If your throat chakra is overactive, you will often be accused of having a loud voice, and you will have a tendency to interrupt others. It may also be possible that you love to hear yourself talk a little too much. An overactive throat chakra can cause a sore throat, mouth ulcers, cavities, and frequent throat infections. If your throat chakra is underactive, you probably have trouble raising your voice and expressing yourself. You act shy around others or pull yourself away from conversations completely. Because unused energy from the throat chakra is usually diverted to the third chakra, an underactive throat chakra can cause digestive problems.

Directly between your eyebrows, you can find your sixth chakra, called the third eye chakra, or Anja. This chakra is associated with psychic powers, as it deals with information beyond the five senses. The sixth chakra helps you find balance and peace with both the material and physical worlds and can help you maintain your faith. It is also the source of good intuition. The third eye chakra is represented by the color purple, though some charts use the color indigo as representation, and it is believed that psychic abilities are developed through this chakra. An overactive third eye chakra is incredibly rare, but in such cases, those with an overactive chakra will find their lives consumed and overwhelmed by paranormal experiences and psychic actions like astrology and tarot reading, that distract them from enjoying the human experience. An underactive third eye chakra is much more common and afflicts the majority of people in the world. An underactive sixth chakra completely cuts you off from all psychic energy and prevents you from receiving any information that does not come from the five senses.

Last is the crown chakra, which is called Sahaswana. It is difficult to explain, but this chakra connects you to the universe and the world around you. The crown chakra is placed at the very top of your head, and your consciousness is hidden somewhere in this chakra. Achieving a balanced crown chakra is extremely difficult, and is similar to the Buddhist concept of reaching nirvana, and is the ultimate goal for all spiritual questors and warriors. This chakra is associated with white, or with clear chakras. Many charts use a dark purple to represent this chakra, as white can be difficult to work with. It is impossible to have an overactive crown chakra, and there is nothing wrong with you if your crown chakra is underused. It just means that you are human.

There are many different ways to throw off the balance within your chakras. From using a chakra too much or too little, to blocking it completely, disrupting the natural flow of the energy coming from your chakras can greatly impact your wellbeing, as well as how you walk through life. It is critical to keep your chakras as healthy and balanced as possible if you want the best life has to offer.

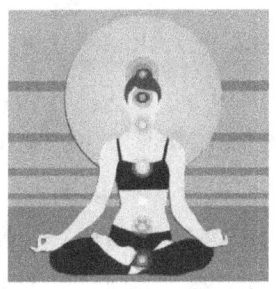

How Crystal Healing Can Help Your Chakras

Chakras provide and control the energy flowing through your body, and crystal healing works through crystals resonating with your natural energy, giving boosts to some types, negating or dampening others, or completely changing how your energy flows and affects you. Thinking like this, it's only natural that crystal healing and chakras go together. Crystals can be a large tool in balancing, cleansing, aligning and unblocking your chakras, as they can help regulate, boost and support the energy of the chakras. Of course, you can't just take any random crystal and start healing. You need to select your stones carefully for each chakra. Luckily there are two simple methods to do that. The first is to choose by purpose and function. Look at the function and purpose of each chakra and choose a crystal with effects that will encourage or boost that purpose, like an amethyst, which boosts spirituality and opens you to the world around you, for your third eye chakra, and malachite, a strong healing crystal, or rose quartz, a crystal that encourages love and affection, for your heart chakra. A crystal with an effect that supports the purpose of the chakra you want to use it with will help strengthen that energy and maintain and continuous flow of that type of energy throughout the body. Another, even easier way, is to choose by color. Looking back a little, you might notice that the general functions and abilities of the different colors of crystals correspond to the functions of the chakra of the same color. Blue crystals help with communication, green crystals heal, and white and clear crystals channel energy and encourage purity. In correspondence, the throat chakra deals with communication and expressing yourself, and is represented with blue; the heart chakra is green, and is the chakra of love, hope, and healing; and the crown chakra is represented by white and is all about connecting to the energy of the world around you. Choosing stones by the colors of your chakras is the quickest and simplest way to choose which crystals to use for healing your chakras. Many crystal stores sell sets of seven crystals that match the colors of the seven chakras called chakra stones. These sets are selected and put together specifically to be used for cleansing and aligning your chakras and are especially useful for beginners.

Now that you know which crystals to use, it's time to learn how to use them. As always, contact and proximity are how this works. Carrying your chakra stones with you is a good idea to get a steady flow of healing energy from them. If you're having trouble with a specific chakra, wear a crystal to help cleanse and strengthen it on you at all times, either in a pocket or purse or as a piece of jewelry. This is a simple way to give basic support to your chakras, but taking the time to have a full healing session can have a much stronger effect. Find somewhere calm and quiet where you can be comfortable and lie down on a soft blanket or carpet. Lie on your back and take a few deep breaths to get calm and relaxed. Place your crystals on your body directly where the chakras are located - the crystal for the crown chakra should be placed on the ground directly above your head, and the root chakra on the ground between your legs. lie there for ten to twenty minutes and let the crystals do their work. Clear your mind and focus on your breathing, or on your chakras and the crystals. Move your thoughts from one chakra to the next and feel the energy flowing through them. Visualize each chakra as a colored wheel of energy turning in a clockwise direction. Let your worries and problems go for a while and let in the healing. After a session like this, you should feel more centered, balanced and relaxed. This method can be used to heal only a few specific chakras, or even just one if it's giving you some serious problems. Just holding a chakra stone near or over your chakra and focusing on its energy can be an easy way to get some quick healing done in a pinch.

It's important to clear your crystals or chakra stones before and after using them to align and balance your chakras. A crystal filled with negative or unwanted energy won't be able to do much to heal your chakras and might throw off its balance even more. You should also make sure your crystals are properly charged, especially the ones you wear as jewelry or carry with you wherever you go. The more you use a crystal, the quicker it loses its energy.

Crystal Healing and Meditation

Meditation is a method of focusing the mind and turning off unnecessary mental chatter. It helps you focus your mind on one specific thought, action, activity or intention. Meditating can help you remove stress from your life, lower your blood pressure and improve spiritual growth. Meditation can also help improve your crystal healing. Meditating on a crystal can help you better connect with its energy and learn to understand it better. Meditation can help you become more in tune with your crystals, and it's a good idea to spend some time meditating with every one of your crystals every now and then. This can help you understand how they work and feel their effects on you much more acutely. You can even have what some call a crystal day, where you spend the whole day meditating with crystals, starting with crystals that have a strong energizing effect. These are usually your red crystals. Move on to orange and yellow and green, working your way through the rainbow until you go from violet to white and finally to clear crystals. This can be an incredible experience that can bring you in tune with the highest possible frequency of crystal vibration and may leave you feeling energized, exalted, and blissed out. It might be a good idea to meditate with a black or brown crystal afterward to ground yourself again. Here is a good exercise to help you meditate with a crystal:

Find a calm, comfortable place where you won't be interrupted, especially by your phone and other people, or distracted by unnecessary things. Again, your phone can be a problem. In fact, just turn off your phone and leave it on the opposite side of your home when you meditate. To start, get yourself settled in a comfortable sitting position and set up your crystal. You can either put it on the floor or a low table in front of you or hold it with both hands in your lap. Focus on your breathing while you let go of all your anxiety and tension. Take a deep breath, making sure that the exhale is just a little longer than the exhale. Breathe in positive and relaxing energy and breathe out all the negativity you have bottled up inside. Keep this up until you've established a slow, steady rhythm. Now shift your focus to your crystal. See its color and shape and feel its weight if you have it in your hands. Feel its vibrations running through you as you study the finer points of the crystal. All the lines and speckles of color. The inner planes and little flaws that make this crystal unique. When you feel you're ready to move on, close your eyes and begin contemplating your crystal. Focus your thoughts on the energy moving into you from the crystal, and let the crystal teach you what it wants you to know about it. This step can be as long or short as you need it to be. When you're finished with your meditation, you can open your eyes again. Plant your feet firmly on the ground and give yourself some time to come back to the present and your body again. Holding a grounding crystal like a smoky quartz or boji stone can help with that.

On the other hand, crystals can help improve your meditation in general. If you're having trouble focusing your mind on the subject of your meditation, having a suitable crystal on you or in the room with you can help focus your mind on where it needs to be. You can either use crystals that improve concentration in general, or you can use a crystal related to what you are meditating on, like using stones like amethyst or lepidolite to assist you when you're meditating for religious reasons or to strengthen your third eye. Or using green crystals when your meditation focuses on healing and growth.

Whether your meditation is focused on your crystals or you're using crystals to enhance your meditation, it's very important to make sure that your crystals are always properly cleansed and have pure energy. Impure energy in a crystal can disrupt your meditation have the opposite effect if you're not careful.

Using Crystals to Improve Your Life

Improving the quality of your life is what crystal healing is all about. From improving your mood to controlling certain elements in your life daily to encourage healing and improving mental stability, there's a crystal that can do it for you, and there are different ways to use these crystals according to what you need.

Combining Crystals and Crystal Healing

Before we get to the various methods of practicing crystal healing, it might be good to know that you can combine crystals with each other for different results. Many crystals have abilities that complement or counter one another, and one crystal likely won't be enough to get all the results out of your crystal healing. Say, for instance, you're having trouble developing your relationship on an emotional level, you could use a rose quartz to boost feelings of love and attraction, and then add an amethyst to dampen the intense physical attraction and raising it to a more spiritual level. Adding a clear quartz to the mix will increase the strength of the impact the crystals have.

Combining different shapes and sizes can help you further narrow down your precise results, as the shape of your crystals have their own effects, and larger crystals have more energy to give than smaller ones.

A wonderful thing about crystal healing is that you can also use it together with other types of healing, medicines, and therapies. Crystals can greatly help improve the results of these healing techniques, and vice versa. Adding essential oils to a crystal massage can do wonders for the mind, body, and spirit.

Wearing Crystals

Wearing crystals is the simplest and most common way of using crystal healing. Crystals emit their own energy constantly, as well as repel and remove other types of energy. By keeping a crystal on your body or in your pocket, that crystal will continue resonating with your energy and you will feel its effects as long as you have it with you. Putting on a crystal necklace or having tumbled stone in your pocket can be compared to taking a vitamin in the morning to nourish you throughout the whole day. Crystal shapes can easily be used to determine exactly what you want to do with your crystal healing, and it's very simple to combine crystals if you want to. The biggest limitation of this method is the size of the crystal. It could become quite tricky to carry a crystal in your coat pocket or tuck it into your bra if it's the size of a tennis ball. Because these crystals tend to be used long term, it's important to regularly clear and charge your crystals to gain the best benefits from them.

Placing Crystals on Your Body

This is the method you use when you want to do something very specific right now. Place your crystal directly where you want its abilities to affect you. This will direct the energy of the crystal directly to the area it's in contact with, and you will feel its effect the strongest in that spot. This method works exactly like applying a balm to a burn or ice to a swollen wrist or ankle. If you feel nauseous, hold a piece of sodalite to your stomach, or if you have a headache, sit down for a while and press a quartz on the spot where the pain is the strongest.

Placing Crystals Around the House

Your home is a very important part of your life, and using crystals is a great way to make your living space a place of safety, serenity, and healing. You can set the charge and mood for each room, helping you build a more perfect home for yourself. You can place barrier crystals at your doors and windows to ward off negative energy and protect your health. Scatter calming and healing crystals around your bathroom to make those long, relaxing baths even better. Put pink crystals in your bedroom to attract romantic energy.

Crystal shapes strongly into play here, as the shape of the crystal can help regulate how the crystal affects the feeling of the room. For example, if you have guests coming over for dinner, us a large round amazonite crystal as a centerpiece. Its ability to encourage communication and truth will be spread evenly all over the room. Scatter a few pieces of tumbled malachite and fluorite around the amazonite to gently radiate a sense of confidence and calmness. Not only will this make a beautiful display and an interesting conversation piece, but it will also help your guests feel confident and relaxed around each other and help them communicate with one another truthfully and with ease.

The same concept can be applied to your car. Simply put a crystal or two, or three or four, on your dashboard, the backseat, the glove compartment, or even the cupholders, and you can receive healing and protection from your crystals as you drive to work or do your shopping.

Sleeping with Crystals

Just because your conscious mind turns off and stops working, doesn't mean your crystals do. There is no reason why you can't receive some crystal healing while you sleep. In fact, it might be even better than when you're awake. When sleeping, your subconscious takes over and you become more susceptible to a crystal's energy. Placing crystals near your bed can help you heal at an accelerated pace while you sleep. They can help you relax before going to bed and protect you from bad dreams and encourage good ones. You should consider which crystals you use carefully. Crystals that improve communication will do you little good in your sleep, and crystals that invigorate you aren't a good idea, but tucking a calming crystal under your pillow can be a great way to fight insomnia.

Crystal Grids

Crystal grids are all about combining crystals and using shapes. Crystal grids are built by placing crystals in a specific geometric shape that has been predetermined. Learning all the different types of grids and how to use them can take a long time, but most are willing to put in the hours, as crystal grids are a very powerful tool. Crystal grids are used to strengthen intention, manifest ambition and greatly enhance the abilities of your crystals. These grids are designed to create especially effective combinations, and the sacred geometries used make your crystals much stronger than they would normally be individually. Crystal grids are also commonly used to enhance spells and form a part of rituals in many cultures and religions. All crystal grids have a larger stone in the center that forms the core of the grid. These are usually pyramids or points to direct and manifest the power, but other shapes can also be used, depending on the purpose of your grid. Next are tumbled and rough stones to form the rest of the grid, and a clear quartz to connect the crystals and activate the grid. Building a grid can be easy to build, but they require a flat surface with enough space for the entire grid. These grids should remain undisturbed, so if you have a cat or a small child, it is important to find a way to keep your grid safe from them. Here are instructions to build a basic crystal grid:

Start with your intention. Decide what you want to do with this grid, and build up from that. You can write down your intention on a piece of paper and leave it folded on the table, or you can just keep it strongly in your thoughts.

Choose a sacred geometry that compliments your intention, as well as all the crystals you are going to use. The crystals should match your intention as much as possible. If you want, you can build your grid on a board and use wire to fix the crystals in place. This can help you keep the crystals on the grid from accidentally being nudged out of place, and you can even have it framed when you're done.

Lay out your crystals according to the grid, starting with the outside and working your way towards the center. Your focal crystal in the middle of the grid should be placed last. Make sure to keep your mind focused on your intention while you work.

Use your clear quartz to connect the points of your grid, again working from the outside inward. Pass your quartz crystal over every single crystal in the grid and keep focussing on your intention.

The final step is to make sure your grid won't be disturbed or disrupted, and feel its powerful effect.

Moving Crystals Around the Body

Crystals don't need to stay in the same place for a long time to make them work. Moving crystals around your body can help spread their energy throughout your body or direct their energy flow more accurately. Removing tension and negative energy all around your body can be very easy with this method. You can move the crystals to where they are needed most, and when they've done their healing work there, you can move on to the next troublesome spot. Wands are a good tool to use here and help direct your energy better and can direct precisely where the energy needs to go or needs to be removed from. Moving the crystals through the air around you can help you cleanse your aura and the energy flowing all around you.

A good example of this method is a crystal massage. This is a technique similar to a hot rock massage, but rather than regular heated stones, different types and shapes of crystals are used. These crystals are chosen according to what you want out of the massage, and different types and shapes are used on the different parts of the body. It's possible to get a full body massage or to focus on a specific area. A crystal massage can be an incredible, divine experience, and, if done right, one single crystal massage can achieve results in one session what might require several sessions of regular massage. Crystal massages can be a great way to achieve perfect balance in the mind, body, and spirit. With a little bit of searching, you can find a professional practitioner to give you one of these massages, but the world is also full of courses and books that can teach you to do this yourself - or to teach a friend how to give you a crystal massage.

It is, of course, important to properly clear your crystals before and after using this method.

Water Infusion

Infusing your drinking water with a crystal's healing energy is a good way to heal and cleanse your body from the inside. Water is good for the body and can carry those healing energies throughout your entire body. Filtering your water through healing stones is a good way to infuse your water, or you could let your water stand for a while with a crystal or two in the glass. You should remove the stones from the glass to prevent accidentally swallowing or choking on a stone. A useful product that is fairly new to the market is a water bottle with a chamber at the bottom where you can lock a healing crystal in place. A more common alternative is to use a water bottle with a built-in infuser usually meant for fruits or herbs. You can freely pick and choose which crystals to use, but be careful around crystals like malachite that are made up of toxic minerals. When infusing your water, it is vital that your crystals are clean of any dirt or bacteria before you use them. Cleansing their energy beforehand is also advised.

Chapter 11: 20 Powerful Crystals And Their Healing Properties

Crystals are increasing in popularity these days, but these old minerals are also old spiritual healing instruments. There are numerous minerals generated in Mother Earth's pressurized womb that rise to the ground to become healing crystals that share their magic and knowledge with us.

Everything surrounding us is made of energy and stones, gems and crystals are no distinct. Each of them is produced up of small crystals in particular molecular structures that are continuously in movement, which also leads each rock and crystal to emit a distinctive vibration and characteristic energy field.

These unique energy vibrations interact with our energetic vibrations and can unequivocally affect us physically, spiritually and sentimentally.

Here Are 20 Powerful Healing Crystals and The Properties They Possess

These antique beauties are here to sustain us and will call us when we require their mending energy. Check out these 20 healing crystals and their characteristics to upgrade your spiritual level and even help you treating physical diseases you may suffer from. Which healing stones are speaking to you?

1. Selenite: The Master

This master mineral classified among the only healing crystals that need not be loaded and may be utilized to clean and recharge other crystals. It is the most common crystal, discovered in old evaporated salt lakes and oceans and can be discovered from Mexico to Brazil and beyond.

Metaphysical healing characteristics: Selenite is a conduit to the greatest point of consciousness and all that is infinite—spirit guides, the cosmos and curiosity. It brings the spiritual world to earth and it reminds us where we come from and where we are going.

Physical curative characteristics: Well-known for its master remedial properties, there's not much that selenite can't be used for. Meditating on the required result and bringing the stone with you can assist deliver excellent healing and inner peace.

2. Moonstone: The Stabilizer

Deeply connected to the female and the moon, the moonstone is the ideal rock to gently generate harmony within and reinforce intuition. It was a rock of divine figures in ancient India and it is considered sacred and royal.

Metaphysical healing characteristics: Moonstone has the ability to open you up to other realms and the Universe itself. It is useful to fight materialism and control the ego, as well.

Physical healing characteristics: Moonstone is utilized to help the pituitary and digestive systems, to fight against obesity, fluid retention, hormonal issues, menstrual issues.

3. Aventurine: The Stone of Opportunity

Recognized for amplifying luck, wealth and abundance, aventurine is a nice rock to bring with you if you're going to play in Las Vegas. Part of the quartz family, this rock draws good luck and helps the effective implementation of fresh possibilities.

Metaphysical healing characteristics: Correlated with the Heart Chakra, this gem can generate a feeling of overall well-being and mental calmness. It harmonizes the mental, physical and spiritual components and restores balance.

Physical healing characteristics: Aventurine supports the flow of the core, blood and energy and can assist speed up regeneration from injury, disease, or surgery.

4. Crystal Quartz: The Spirit Stone

Probably the most well-known gemstone, crystal quartz is viewed as a speck of light into the abstract world.

Metaphysical healing characteristics: this specific crystal includes the full spectrum of colors and can be easily utilized to augment wishes, rituals and manifestations from the nonphysical world to the physical one. Meditate on the glass and "program" the crystal with your wishes. Then you can wear or bring your crystal anywhere to amplify your energy and boost the manifestation of your wishes.

Physical healing characteristics: Crystal glass is a supreme healer and is believed to boost immunity and the circulatory systems and rise the flow of qi energy into the body.

5. Citrine: The Money Stone

The sort of quartz, the golden yellow color of this crystal, is connected with its association to cash, gold and prosperity.

Metaphysical healing characteristics: take this stone with you to the bank, to company conferences concerning finances, or put citrine on your table and look at it while you operate. Citrine can assist you gain riches and financial wealth and stabilization.

Physical healing characteristics: Citrine is considered to boost metabolism and support digestion and nausea. It is also possible to use it to reinforce nerve impulses, assisting the brain in burning more quickly and strongly.

6. Agate: Stone of Inner Stability

This diverse stone can be discovered in almost all colors with a big variety of striations. From clear transparent, stained and highly striped, agate personifies our inner nature.

Metaphysical healing characteristics: Agate increases self-awareness, stabilizes the aura (in all its colors), converts adverse energy and is a strong driving force of the spirit. Use this stone to cure frustration, mental disturbance and absence of self-worth.

Physical healing characteristics: Known for enhancing mental function by enhancing the clarity of thought, agate is a fantastic rock that you can utilize before a significant exam, when composing, or when collecting ideas for significant discussion with someone you enjoy and want to interact effectively with.

7. Tourmaline: The Grounding Stone

Tourmaline, the preferred talisman of protection, is used as a psychic shield to base your energy and fight the introduction of adverse forces into your energy domain. Long used by sorcerers, shamans, witches and magicians, tourmaline can be discovered on every continent.

Metaphysical healing characteristics: Although tourmaline is a deep black, it can be used to remove adverse emotions, increase your vibration and bring you into the sun. Black absorbs light as it functions as a sponge for damaging or dark materials. It promotes you to stay radiant in dark moments.

Physical healing characteristics: use tourmaline to relieve pain in the joints and help to re-align the spine. It can also be used to reinforce the immune system, the heart and the adrenal cells–relaxing pressure and relaxing tension.

8. Rose Quartz: The Love Stone

This lovely purple quartz is connected with the core and expresses unconditional love for oneself, others and the planet.

Metaphysical healing characteristics: a marvelous stone that invites you to love, helps you to give love or attract a soulmate, rose quartz is all about the core. Wear or wear rose quartz to open up to discovering happiness if you're single and to deepen and nurture your love if you're in a partnership.

Physical healing characteristics: centered around the heart Chakra, this gemstone is useful for profound mental bonding and discharge and is known to enhance flow and reduced blood pressure. It is potentially helpful in relieving palpitations or missed beats and stress.

9. Turquoise: The Protection Stone

Believed to be the most antique gem known to humankind, turquoise has always been cherished by leaders, shamans, rulers, wizards and suchlike. Know as a sign of wisdom, turquoise is common in almost all old societies and has always been regarded as the rock of safety.

Metaphysical healing characteristics: Turquoise strengthens the intuition and meditation. It is also connected with the Throat Chakra, which promotes transparent communication, due to its black hue. Carry turquoise as a charm of safety and as a channel of old wisdom.

Physical healing characteristics: Assisting in mental issues, neck or ear pain and throat disfunctions, turquoise is very much linked with the psychic domain, making it an excellent rock to clear blockages and promote a good stream of energy throughout the body.

10. Fluorite: The Stone of Positivity

Perhaps this crystal is among the most underrated, but at the same time one of the strongest. This rock is regarded to pull adverse energy and small temperatures out of space or your body and to make room for the sun to shine in. Found in various color variants, fluorite is a magical crystal.

Metaphysical healing characteristics: used to protect the auric, increase your vibration, alchemize adverse energy and soothe a messy mind. Rainbow Fluorite is better known for stabilizing the mind and amplifying the psychic link and enhancing intuitive capabilities.

Physical healing characteristics: this vibrant rock can be used when learning to release your mind and sharpen your concentration. It is also useful to relieve body swelling, to dissipate cold diseases and to cure mucous membrane.

11. Lapis Lazuli: The Stone of Truth

This lovely, blue glass is among the most dynamic, old and sought-after crystals on earth. It has long been connected with royalty and luxury and its heavenly characteristics help the ones in the physical realm with wisdom and excellent judgment.

Metaphysical healing characteristics: Lapis Lazuli activates celestial upper Chakras and enables the Throat Chakra to communicate clearly and express one's thoughts easily. This fascinating stone encourages internal reflection and reality as it helps the exploration and depiction of the spirit realm.

Physical healing characteristics: use this strong stone to support and cure the neck, larynx and vocal cords. Because of its powerful links to the brain, it is thought to relieve Attention Deficit Disorder (ADD) by assisting the mind to concentrate and release useless thoughts.

12. Hematite: The Grounding Stone

This iron-rich rock is deeply grounded and linked to the earth. Mostly known as the "bloodstone" in ancient Greece because of the black hue of the iron material discovered in nature.

Metaphysical healing characteristics: Hematite directly affects the Root Chakra and possesses a deeply grounded energy that emphasizes our natural life and promotes us socially.

Physical healing characteristics: the iron discovered in hepatitis can assist us clean the blood, enhance circulation, handle uneven menstrual flow and promote a good body. It was also proven to be useful in liberating stress and anxiety and calming the nervous system.

13. Jade: The Dream Stone

This is another vibrant rock that can be discovered in a vast range of colors, worldwide. The region dictates the color and this stone is one of the most used. It has been celebrated across societies, centuries and millennia (and into contemporary times) for its physical and metaphysical healing characteristics, placing it among the most popular crystals known to man.

Metaphysical healing characteristics: jade reflects the nobleness of status and values. This rock is also linked to the core and enables us to acknowledge the reality, to communicate love (self and others) and to access the shamanic worlds in a dream state.

Physical healing characteristics: given the strong bond with the nucleus, Jade is useful for reducing toxins and purifying the body as a whole through the blood. It is also useful in relieving joint pain and speeding up the recovery process after surgeries.

14. Amethyst: The Manifestation Stone

Besides selenite and crystal quartz, it is one of the most encountered rocks in the New Age. Amethyst is present in a form or another everywhere on the globe. This lovely purple crystal is well recognized for many things, but the demonstration is the most important among the characteristics.

Metaphysical healing characteristics: connect with amethyst to your heart's wishes and life's intent and then express it in your life! This strong crystal is connected with the upper Chakras, assisting us in taking the etheric domain to the physical plane. This involves bringing to life our earthly dreams.

Physical healing characteristics: use amethyst to increase the sympathetic nervous system, equilibrium hormones, alleviate headaches, ease the stress in the throat and treat insomnia. Place the amethyst under your pillow at night to ensure that you can sleep profoundly and wake up relaxed, prepared to produce and communicate.

15. Kyanite: The Stone of Emotion

Kyanite helps the mind to build connections where none existed before, particularly in terms of mental growth and meditation. It does not collect adverse energy, so it does not need to be cleaned and can effectively be used to purify other rocks and rooms. The soothing blue-green tone is connected with the heavens and is therefore highly relaxing and nerve-friendly.

Metaphysical healing characteristics: Psychic skills can be improved by cyanite as it deepens meditation and connects pathways to the spirit realm. It might also help assisting those who are transitioning through death.

Physical healing characteristics: Cyanite is great to assist cure any pain in the neck and enhance communication. It is wonderful to relieve headaches, eye pain from looking at a laptop and neck strain.

16. Obsidian: The Mirror Stone

The jet-black rock is a mirror rock because of its capacity to improve the vision and the manner you see the universe and the situations. It's an extremely reflective surface and coherent coloring allow you to look profoundly inside to uncover your soul and the healing needed to raise your vibration.

Metaphysical healing properties: the use of the obsidian goes back to the Stone Age and its natural characteristics have been understood to allow the vision of other beings, of the soul itself and of places not available from the land, to achieve wisdom and understanding. Use this rock to disclose your shadows, faults and weaknesses in order to better comprehend yourself.

Physical healing characteristics: use obsidian to relieve emotional distress that has long been buried, overlooked, or even erased from memory. It is also a great remedy to relieve pressure and anxiety connected with mental trauma.

17. Blue Topaz: The Stone of Creativity

The light green color of the topaz represents the mind and our creative ability. It can assist boost the mind to learn more rapidly and to maintain data that can be used for years to come. It is also helpful in creating creativity and opening the mind to fresh thoughts.

Metaphysical healing qualities: since Topaz is a rock of the mind, it is good to connect with one's angels, spirit guides and close people whom you've lost. Use the topaz to expand your mind, open your soul and align yourself with the spirit realm.

Physical healing characteristics: Topaz has long been considered to help with mental illness, eye disease, dimness in vision and to recover loss of flavor.

18. Opal: The Eye Stone

This wonderful and colorful rock appears to be on fire with a rainbow spectrum of electrical colors as it moves in the sun. It's directly connected to the eye as it is so enjoyable to look at and linked with the pineal gland (Third Eye Chakra).

Conclusion

Thank you again for reading this book! I hope this book was able to help you to understand and get to know this alternative way of healing better. Often times, alternative medicine and healing procedures are neglected by the medical community mainly because most of these products and therapies lack the necessary scientific and medical proof that most synthetic drugs have. They also usually laughed at because most scientists and medical practitioners call them as pseudoscience. They say that these alternative means of healing do not have enough scientific proof and basis, therefore they are inferior to the commercial and synthetic drugs that pharmaceuticals produce.

However, what most people don't realize is that these alternative medicines and therapeutic procedures, such as crystal healing, totally safe and natural ways of healing that are effective in making our health problems go away in just an affordable amount. You really have nothing to lose if you consider trying these alternative healing cures for your health problems. Just remember to always research first and now as much as you can about these alternative medicines because knowledge is power, always, and knowing something ahead of time can sometimes spell the difference between life and death.

I also hope that through reading this book, you were able to understand the basic concepts and techniques used in the art of healing through therapeutic crystals. I hope that you were able to grasp the essence of this alternative healing therapy and legitimately understood what it can really do for you and for others. The steps and techniques that were taught in this book were practically very easy to follow and try. Hopefully, you also learned by heart the different kinds of crystals, the different groups that they belong to and when to appropriately use the crystals in each color group in order to heal different kinds of illnesses. I also look forward to the fulfillment of my expectation that you were able to comprehend the concept of chakras and their importance.

I hope you were encouraged to practice, try and learn more about the art of crystal healing and use the knowledge that you were able to acquire from this book as a stepping stone into making yourself a certified crystal healer and an expert in this craft.

The next step upon successful completion of this book is to of course practice and apply what you have learned. Practice and application always go hand in hand in retaining the information that one has learned. Without practice, the skills that you learned from this book will never be enhanced and be cultivated. Try to quiz yourself if you really know the uses of the different crystals. Try to match the sickness with the appropriate crystals that can cure them. Try to find the location of your chakra without looking at a guide. Try the simple and different ways of cleansing your crystals. Try and try and practice until you have mastered the craft of crystal healing because that will be the only true way of succeeding.

May you also pass on to others the techniques and the knowledge about the art of crystal healing that you have learned in this book so that you can inspire others to learn and appreciate this kind of alternative therapy as much as this book has encouraged and inspired you to look into this bizarre but surely interesting therapeutic procedure. Remember as well to always learn and learn no matter how knowledgeable you become in crystal healing for there will always be new and available information, waiting for you to discover. A great crystal healer will never stop researching and learning all about his or her craft.

www.ingramcontent.com/pod-product-compliance
Lightning Source LLC
Chambersburg PA
CBHW071828080526
44589CB00012B/945